# Rekindling Desire

## A Guide to Restoring Male Libido

By
Dr. Daniel A. Harlow

# Rekindling Desire

## A Guide to Restoring Male Libido

# Table of Contents

# Chapter 1:
## Introduction

In the labyrinth of modern life, it's easy for many men to find themselves quietly grappling with a decline in sexual desire. This journey we're embarking upon delves into an issue as ancient as it is perennial, buoyed by complexity, and shrouded in a silence that's rarely broken. But it's not just about the immediate loss of libido. It's about that sweeping introspection, the conflicts it ushers into relationships, and the undreamt-of potential lying dormant beneath misunderstood concerns.

For many men, the shifting tides of sexual desire can feel intensely personal and sometimes isolating. There is an inherent societal pressure to remain stoic, a fortress of masculinity and virility. Yet, when desire wanes, the silence in its wake can amplify feelings of inadequacy and self-doubt. These experiences, though personal, are far from unique. In seeking to address this silent epidemic, we aim to create a compassionate dialogue that fosters understanding and hope.

Understanding libido loss demands more than a cursory glance at physical health or obvious societal influences. It's a comprehensive exploration that intertwines physical, emotional, and relational domains. The foundation of this discourse is to arm men and their partners with the necessary tools and knowledge, empowering them to regain not just their libido but a deeper connection with themselves and each other. Our journey will traverse varied terrains—from exploring hormonal influences and lifestyle choices to examining the psychological underpinnings that hold sway over one's libido.

Intimacy, in its most authentic form, exists when partners are open about their vulnerabilities and fears. When communicating freely, examining inhibitions, and jointly seeking resolution, relationships don't just survive—they thrive. It's about creating a bridge built on trust, empathy, and shared aspirations. This book will act as a spade to dig deep into these concepts, giving readers the confidence and ability to nurture those crucial connections.

What we offer isn't a mere collection of abstract ideas. It's a call to action framed around real-world implications. Men need to recognise that experiences of libido change aren't solely theirs to bear. They're shared both with partners who notice changes in intimacy and desire and with communities that benefit when individuals feel understood and supported.

The word "libido" carries heavy connotations. For those facing dips in sexual desire, it can seem like a contrived reality demanding correction or disguise. Here, though, we aspire to remove the stigma, replacing it with stories of resilience and revitalisation. Because at the heart of every challenge lies the opportunity for growth and transformation.

Consider this introduction a gentle invitation to dive deeper. The following chapters promise a fertile ground of insights and strategies that aim to alleviate stress, improve mental health, and adapt lifestyle changes conducive to enhanced libido. We'll confront myths, dissect complexities, and provide a roadmap towards rekindled passion, stability, and improved sexual wellness.

As we proceed, remember this is not some clinical narrative or a detached analysis of libido loss. We recognise the reality of what men endure and, importantly, what their partners experience too. The goal is to breathe life back into these relationships by providing clarity and practical steps, enlivened with motivational and inspirational undertones to encourage proactive engagement.

Libido doesn't operate in a vacuum. Our examination begins with this expansive introduction and continues to tap into individual nuances. Each chapter will tackle distinct yet interrelated components affecting desire. Whether it's the interplay of hormonal shifts or the weight of societal pressure affecting psychological health, each aspect interweaves with the next, painting a holistic picture where clarity eclipses confusion.

With empathy as our guide, this journey is also about opening new pathways for dialogue. The concepts explored will not only present solutions but equip readers with the vocabulary and confidence needed to express concerns and strategies with their partners. It's about engendering confidence, fostering connection, and ensuring that each person involved feels valued and understood.

In the end, our aim is for you to emerge with a robust understanding of libido dynamics, arming you with the insights necessary to revitalise these fundamental aspects of your being. While the future chapters will build upon this foundation, weaving in detailed dissections of various influences, it is the spirit of this introduction that sets the tone: one of exploration, honesty, and enduring hope.

# Chapter 2:
# Understanding Male Libido

In the labyrinth of human sexuality, male libido plays a pivotal role, one that intertwines both body and mind in a dance of desire and vitality. It is not merely a biological impulse but a tapestry woven with threads of psychological and physical factors that collectively impact a man's drive for intimacy. Understanding male libido requires peering beyond the simple mechanics of arousal, delving into the heart of what stirs passion and what causes it to wane. Each individual's journey through libido fluctuations can feel personal, yet it is a shared experience influenced by a myriad of factors like stress, health, and emotional connectivity. By unpacking these elements, we aim to dispel myths, foster awareness, and inspire proactive steps towards revitalising one's sexual essence. This chapter serves as a cornerstone in recognising the nuances of male desire, empowering men and their partners to forge stronger, more fulfilling connections. Recognising the significance of libido in overall well-being illuminates not only the path of self-awareness but also offers a beacon of hope for rekindling the flame of intimacy.

## Causes of Decline

When it comes to understanding male libido, it's vital to acknowledge the factors that can lead to its decline. It's a multifaceted issue that doesn't just stem from one clear cause. Instead, it's a tapestry woven from your physical health, psychological well-being, and the dynamics of your close relationships. Unraveling this complex subject requires insight into the myriad influences at play.

One of the primary causes of decreased libido is stress. In today's fast-paced world, stress creeps in from every corner, whether it be work, finances, or family responsibilities. This chronic state of tension isn't just a mental burden; it can have cascading effects on your body's hormonal balance, particularly on testosterone levels. Stress triggers the release of cortisol, a hormone that can lower testosterone, leading to a reduction in sexual desire. It's a vicious cycle that you may not even be fully aware of, yet it impacts your intimate life profoundly.

Physical health issues are another prevalent reason for the decline in libido. Conditions such as obesity, diabetes, and cardiovascular diseases can directly influence your ability to maintain sexual interest and performance. These ailments don't just zap your energy; they can also alter your body's hormonal milieu, further dampening desire. Tackling these health challenges requires a holistic approach, integrating lifestyle changes with medical interventions where necessary.

Consider also the inevitable passage of time. Ageing brings with it hormonal changes that can contribute to a diminished sex drive. Testosterone levels in men naturally decrease as they age, which can affect libido. While this is a normal part of the ageing process, it doesn't mean giving up on a fulfilling intimate life. Understanding these changes and adapting your lifestyle and expectations accordingly is crucial to maintaining a vibrant sexual connection with your partner.

Psychological factors play a crucial role as well. Mental health issues such as depression and anxiety are notorious libido killers. When your mind is clouded by worry or weighed down by the heaviness of depression, sexual desire can take a backseat. These conditions often create a sense of disconnect not only from your partner but also from your own body, adding to the challenge. Seeking professional help and adopting mental health strategies can be transformative and bring a renewed sense of vitality and desire.

Relationship dynamics shouldn't be underestimated in their effect on libido. The emotional bond between you and your partner serves as the foundation for sexual interest and satisfaction. Conflict, lack of communication, and unresolved issues can simmer just below the surface, dampening desire. Emphasising open dialogue, mutual respect, and emotional intimacy can reignite not only passion but also the connection that fuels it.

Substance use and lifestyle choices also make a significant impact. Excessive alcohol consumption, smoking, and drug use have all been linked to reduced libido. These substances can affect circulation, energy levels, and hormonal balance, which in turn can inhibit sexual function and interest. Evaluating and adjusting these habits may be essential steps in restoring a healthy sex drive.

Lastly, misconceptions about male sexuality may indirectly contribute to a decline in libido. Cultural narratives often paint men as perpetually ready and willing, which can create immense pressure and unrealistic expectations. When personal reality doesn't match these portrayals, it can lead to feelings of inadequacy and anxiety, further suppressing libido. Education and open conversations about these misconceptions can help relieve pressure and foster a healthier understanding of one's own desires and capacities.

In summary, while the decline of male libido can be distressing, understanding the multitude of factors involved is the first step towards addressing it. Whether it's through managing stress, improving physical health, strengthening emotional bonds with a partner, or correcting harmful lifestyle choices, it's essential to approach this issue with empathy and knowledge. It's not merely about reclaiming lost desire, but about fostering overall well-being and connection. With patience and the right tools, you can navigate these challenges and kindle the flame of intimacy in your relationship once more.

## Psychological Factors

When we explore the complex realm of male libido, it becomes crucial to delve into the intricate psychological factors that can significantly influence sexual desire. At its core, libido is as much a psychological phenomenon as it is a biological one. The mind's role in regulating sexual desire is pivotal, acting as both a facilitator and barrier, depending on various psychological elements involved.

One of the primary psychological influences on libido is an individual's self-perception and self-esteem. The way a man perceives himself can either energise or debilitate his sexual desire. A negative self-image can lead to feelings of inadequacy, which, in turn, creates a barrier to sexual desire. Conversely, a healthy self-esteem often correlates with a more robust libido. Feeling confident and comfortable in one's own skin is an empowering force, fuelling passion and sexual expression without restraint.

Additionally, past experiences and emotional baggage play substantial roles in shaping current sexual desire. Traumatic experiences or relationships in the past can create subconscious blocks, leading to anxiety or aversion related to sexual activity. Even without overt trauma, negative past encounters can influence expectations and trigger fears of repeating undesirable outcomes. Overcoming these barriers often requires introspection and, at times, professional guidance.

Stress, an all-too-common aspect of modern life, can also suppress libido significantly. The pressures of work, family obligations, and financial concerns can weigh heavily on the mind, diminishing the mental energy required for a healthy libido. The psychological toll of stress often manifests physically, making it difficult for individuals to engage in and enjoy sexual activities. Finding effective stress-management strategies is crucial in mitigating its impact on one's sex life.

Moreover, the interplay between mood disorders and sexual desire is another critical psychological factor. Conditions such as depression and anxiety can severely dampen libido. These conditions don't merely steal energy and joy from daily activities; they also rob individuals of their desire for intimacy and connection. Often, the medications prescribed to treat these conditions might further impact libido, creating a unique challenge that needs careful management.

Emotional intimacy—or the lack thereof—also plays a vital role. A fulfilling sexual relationship is typically rooted in a strong emotional connection. When partners share a deep emotional bond, it often translates into a more vibrant and rewarding sexual relationship. Conversely, unresolved conflict, resentment, or a lack of emotional closeness could elevate stress levels and reduce sexual interest, sometimes creating a vicious cycle of disconnection.

Cultural and societal norms surrounding masculinity and sexuality can impose additional psychological burdens. Men often feel undue pressure to conform to specific ideals regarding sexual prowess and frequency. These unrealistic standards can lead to performance anxiety and self-doubt, clouding the natural ebb and flow of sexual desire with performance pressures. Deconstructing these societal expectations can relieve some of the psychological weight impeding one's libido.

Cognitive habits, often unconscious, play a part as well. Negative thinking patterns, such as catastrophising or holding onto limiting beliefs about one's sexual worth or capabilities, can have a profound impact. These thoughts can create anticipation of failure or rejection, thus creating a self-fulfilling prophecy. Ultimately, breaking free from these patterns through techniques like cognitive restructuring can help restore healthy sexual desire.

Another aspect to consider is the power of mindfulness and presence during intimate moments. Being fully present can enhance pleasurable experiences and deepen connections between partners. Distractions from digital devices or wandering thoughts about daily hassles can sideline intimacy. Practices that cultivate mindfulness can remind individuals to focus on and savour their interactions, fostering a more fulfilling sexual experience.

The stigma surrounding discussions about mental and sexual health can prevent men from seeking the help they need. Fear of being perceived as weak or dysfunctional might lead individuals to suppress their issues, amplifying feelings of isolation. Encouraging open and non-judgmental dialogues about these experiences can be a healing process, reducing the psychological burden significantly.

Ultimately, the psychological terrain of male libido is complex and multifaceted. Understanding these psychological factors can empower men and their partners to address challenges with compassion and determination. By acknowledging these influences and working towards resolving them, individuals can reclaim their sexual vitality and enrich their intimate relationships. Taking steps towards building a supportive psychological framework can reignite passion and foster deeper, more meaningful connections.

## Physical Influences

A decline in male libido might be shrouded in mystery for many, yet, when we peel back the layers, we find physical influences playing a crucial role. It's not unusual for men to experience a drop in sexual desire as they go through different phases of life. Understanding how physical factors impact libido can be empowering, providing pathways to revitalise this vital part of one's life.

To start, let's consider the role of fitness and health. An active lifestyle doesn't just enhance overall well-being; it's also closely tied to sexual health. Regular exercise improves cardiovascular function, which is essential for a healthy sex drive. Good circulation is the backbone of sexual response, ensuring that blood flow reaches the areas it's needed most. Moreover, staying fit can enhance stamina and energy levels, vital components in maintaining an active libido.

However, it's not just about how much you move; what you eat also weighs heavily on your libido. A balanced diet rich in fruits, vegetables, lean proteins, and healthy fats can bolster sexual desire. Essential nutrients, including zinc, selenium, and certain vitamins, have been shown to positively affect hormone levels, which are critical in the orchestration of sexual health.

A frequent yet often overlooked contributor to libido fluctuation is medication. Many common prescription drugs can affect sexual desire, sometimes in unpredictable ways. While they may be indispensable for treating certain health conditions, it's crucial to recognise potential side effects related to sexual function. Open communication with a healthcare provider can facilitate the tweaking of medication to better accommodate sexual health requirements.

Another physical aspect intertwined with libido is sleep quality. Sufficient and restful sleep is non-negotiable for maintaining hormonal balance, particularly testosterone, which is a key driver of male libido. Sleep disorders or consistently poor sleep can disrupt this balance, leading to a noticeable decrease in sexual interest. Balancing work, rest, and relaxation can often yield remarkable improvements in both energy levels and sexual desire.

Furthermore, chronic health conditions such as diabetes, hypertension, or obesity may significantly impact libido. These ailments often come with physiological changes that can impair sexual function. For instance, high blood pressure can damage the arteries, limiting blood flow needed for erections. Managing these conditions through medical treatment and lifestyle adjustments can, therefore, make a drastic difference, not only to general health but also to private life.

Sometimes, the strain of a physically demanding job can also take a toll on libido. Occupations that require prolonged periods of physical exertion or irregular hours can lead to fatigue and stress, both of which are libido dampeners. Striking a balance between work commitments and personal well-being is essential for sustained desire and intimacy.

Age naturally brings about changes in physical condition, including a gradual decline in certain hormone levels. Testosterone levels, for example, tend to decrease with age, influencing the sex drive. Nevertheless, many men find that with age comes the benefit of experience and a deeper emotional connection with their partners, which can enhance the quality of intimacy even if the frequency changes.

Then there are the external environments that play a subtle, yet significant role in shaping one's sexual desire. Pollutants, stressors, and exposure to endocrine-disrupting chemicals can negatively impact libido. Being conscious of environmental factors and making lifestyle choices that minimise exposure to harmful substances can support better sexual health.

Exploring these physical influences is pivotal in understanding the ebb and flow of male libido. Acknowledging that multiple factors can intersect and affect sexual desire encourages a comprehensive strategy to address and improve it. By proactively managing physical health, men can reclaim control over their libido, eventually transforming the journey into one of personal discovery and improved relational harmony.

In recognising that a multitude of physical influences shape male libido, men and their partners are better equipped to navigate this journey. This journey involves understanding the physical wisdom of the body, making informed choices, and developing habits that nurture sexual vitality. Ultimately, this knowledge empowers men not just to overcome barriers to desire but to ignite a deeper connection with themselves and their partners in the process.

# Chapter 3:
## The Role of Hormones

As we delve deeper into understanding the intricate dynamics of male libido, it becomes clear that hormones play a pivotal role in shaping our desires and responses. Consider testosterone—often dubbed the "hormone of desire"—which significantly influences libido. As men age, hormonal balances naturally shift, sometimes leading to a decline in sexual desire. However, these hormonal changes aren't solely dictated by age; lifestyle factors and health conditions can also tip the scales. Embracing the complexities of our hormonal landscape can be empowering. By recognising and addressing these shifts, men and their partners can foster a deeper connection and find pathways to rekindle intimacy, defying the misconceptions that ageing inevitably dampens passion. Understanding this landscape is not just about reclaiming lost desires, but also about enhancing overall well-being and vitality. Through awareness and proactive strategies, the journey towards revitalised intimacy becomes an achievable goal, resonating with hope and resilience.

## Testosterone's Impact

In the tapestry of male biology, testosterone weaves critical threads that influence not only physical appearance and strength but also sexual desire, a subject close to the heart of many. This hormone serves as a barometer of male libido, steering not just physical drive but also contributing to mental vigour and emotional connection.

Understanding testosterone's impact is akin to deciphering a key chapter in the story of male vitality.

Testosterone, often associated with the quintessential elements of masculinity, orchestrates an array of bodily functions. It affects fat distribution, red blood cell production, and bone density, but perhaps its role as a major determinant of sexual health garners most attention. For many men, testosterone levels and sexual desire famously travel in tandem. A decline in this hormone, therefore, can correspond with waning libido, inviting not just a physical void but emotional and relational shifts. It's crucial to see testosterone not as an isolated player but part of a hormonal symphony that balances emotional, psychological, and physical aspects of sex.

While testosterone levels naturally fluctuate throughout life, they typically peak during adolescence and early adulthood, bestowing energy, confidence, and of course, a robust libido. However, as men age, a gradual decline in testosterone production is common, often leading to distinct changes. Such hormonal shifts, subtle at first, can lead to noticeable alterations in libido, making sexual encounters less frequent or less desired. It's like a once-clear radio signal becoming plagued by static — the desire is there, but the clarity seems missing.

Reports and studies continue to delve into the precise impact of testosterone levels on male libido. While testosterone isn't the sole determinant of sexual interest, it undeniably plays a weighty role. Its decline doesn't only affect sexual activity frequency but can also alter sexual satisfaction and performance. Men may find themselves on an emotionally challenging terrain, compelled to unravel the mysteries behind a faltering libido.

This reduction in testosterone levels might manifest through more than just diminished sexual desire. Fatigue, a drop in motivation, and mood changes can cloak the real cause, leaving both partners puzzled. Communication might become strained as frustration mounts, leading to misunderstandings or even relational distance. Recognising hormonal shifts as contributors to these changes is essential, offering not just clarity but paving the way for compassionate dialogue.

It's important to acknowledge that testosterone's impact extends beyond the sheets. As testosterone levels dip, self-esteem might take a hit, and the confidence that once came effortlessly might now require conscious effort. Such is the intertwined nature of testosterone and male psyche; impacts are more layered than they initially appear. The linkage between hormone levels and intimacy encapsulates both physiological and psychological realms, underscoring why both partners might feel its ebb.

Fortunately, there are holistic approaches to managing these hormonal fluctuations. Lifestyle changes such as maintaining a balanced diet, regular physical activity, and quality sleep have shown promising results in supporting healthy testosterone levels. These strategies offer a way to take control, to invite proactive steps, and to counter the hormonal tide.

Furthermore, seeking medical advice for hormone replacement therapy or other interventions can furnish a viable path for some. It's a journey from questioning to understanding to action, aimed at preserving and sometimes reigniting the vibrant flame of desire. Each step, driven by awareness and willingness to adapt, marks progress towards living more fully and reconnecting intimately.

But it's not just about settling for a solution; it's about viewing this as an opportunity for growth. Embracing these changes together, couples can build resilience and deepen their emotional bonds. It offers a fresh perspective on intimacy, one that values emotional vulnerability alongside physical connection.

So, in exploring testosterone's influence, there lies an invitation to greater self-awareness and deeper relational dynamics. It's less about reclaiming something lost and more about adapting to new rhythms, redefining intimacy to fit the contours of these changes. Through understanding testosterone's role, men and their partners illuminate new pathways to intimacy, aligning biology with the shared journey of passion and connection.

## Hormonal Imbalances

Hormones are complex messengers that wield hefty power in our bodies. Imagine them as the conductors of a grand orchestra, orchestrating everything from our mood to our metabolism. When they work in harmony, life can feel like a well-composed symphony, but when they fall out of balance, the discord can be profound. For men navigating a decline in sexual desire, understanding hormonal imbalances is crucial. It's not just about testosterone; it's a complex interplay of various hormones that, when disrupted, can lead to challenges in maintaining intimacy.

**Testosterone** is often centre stage when we discuss male libido. It's no secret that this androgen is pivotal in driving sexual desire. However, it's vital to look beyond testosterone alone, as other hormones, such as estrogen, prolactin, and thyroid hormones, are also significant players in this delicate ecosystem. When any of these hormones veer off course, it can result in imbalances that have repercussions on even day-to-day levels of desire.

Let's delve into how these imbalances might manifest. Low testosterone, or *hypogonadism*, can lead to a reduced interest in sexual activity, fatigue, and even mood swings. But it's not just about having enough testosterone; maintaining the right balance between testosterone and estrogen is crucial. A rise in estrogen levels, for instance, can lead to a decrease in libido since this can affect testosterone's availability and activity in the body.

One contributing factor to hormonal imbalance is **prolactin**. Typically associated with lactation, high levels of prolactin in men can suppress testosterone production and promote erectile dysfunction, both of which are decidedly unhelpful when trying to rekindle the flames of desire. Stress and certain medications might increase prolactin levels, making it a significant player in the hormonal landscape of libido.

You shouldn't overlook the **thyroid**, either. This butterfly-shaped powerhouse in your neck is responsible for releasing hormones that regulate your metabolism. Both hyperthyroidism (excess of thyroid hormone) and hypothyroidism (deficiency of thyroid hormone) can lead to reduced sexual interest and performance, highlighting the interconnectedness of our body systems. A well-tuned thyroid supports optimal energy levels and can significantly influence sexual health indirectly.

Aging also tends to throw a spanner into the works. As we age, hormonal production changes naturally, and this can exacerbate minor imbalances present earlier in life. It's part of the reason why you might notice libido waning as years go by. Yet, with the appropriate knowledge and guidance, these changes don't necessarily spell the end of passion.

It's easy to feel overwhelmed when faced with the intricacy of hormonal imbalances, but fear not; understanding is the first step to overcoming. The key lies in recognising the signs and seeking professional advice. Simple blood tests can help pinpoint which hormones might be causing trouble, guiding strategies that can help restore harmony.

Moreover, lifestyle plays a huge role in hormonal balance. Diet, sleep, stress levels, and even exercise routines contribute to the way our body manages and produces these vital chemical messengers. Regular physical activity, for instance, can boost testosterone and improve mood by regulating serotonin levels, which might help counteract some of the imbalances experienced.

However, don't mistake quick fixes as panaceas. While certain supplements and dietary changes may offer support, it's about consistency. Sustainable lifestyle changes that foster good hormonal health should be the goal, and they may just be the kickstart needed for those struggling with libido issues.

If you're facing the frustrating reality of hormonal imbalances, you're not alone. The path forward involves identifying which hormones need addressing and finding holistic strategies that suit you. Hormonal therapy might sometimes be necessary, but often, small changes in lifestyle and diet can make large strides in improving balance.

Proactivity is empowering. Recognising the role that hormonal imbalances play not only shines a light on the underlying causes of libido loss but also equips you with the tools to address them. As you learn more, you can begin to design a life that not only reignites desire but also enriches your overall sense of well-being.

The journey to understanding hormonal imbalances isn't solely about restoring what once was. It's also about discovery and adaptation, leading to a more profound connection with yourself and others. Although hormones may seem elusive, they ultimately hold the key to navigating many aspects of our lives, including the tender, intimate parts that connect us to our partners.

## Age and Hormonal Changes

Our journey through life is marked by numerous transitions, and the evolution of our hormonal landscape is an undeniable part of this journey. Hormones, those intricate chemical messengers, orchestrate a symphony within our bodies that dictates everything from mood to energy levels. As we age, this symphony begins to shift its pace and rhythm, bringing with it a cascade of changes, particularly in relation to sexual health and desire.

Men, much like their female counterparts, experience significant hormonal shifts over time. A key player in this drama is testosterone, the hormone often heralded as the cornerstone of male vitality and libido. From around the age of thirty, a man's testosterone levels typically begin to decline gradually, a process that medical professionals refer to as 'andropause.' However, not all changes are identical; they are as individual as the men experiencing them.

*Understanding these changes is crucial for both men and their partners, as it offers not only insight but also a foundation for empathy and proactive management.* As testosterone levels drop, men might notice a decrease in energy, mood fluctuations, and a reduced interest in sex. These symptoms can be strikingly similar to those experienced by women during menopause, although they tend to occur more gradually. While the term 'male menopause' has been coined, it's not entirely accurate as the hormonal transition in men is much less abrupt.

Importantly, lower testosterone isn't solely responsible for changes in libido. The body is an interdependent system, and other hormonal players, such as oestrogen, surprisingly play a role even in men. As testosterone levels decrease, the conversion of testosterone to oestrogen might increase, adding to the complex hormonal milieu. This shift doesn't signal a loss of masculinity but rather underscores the intricate balance our bodies strive to maintain.

But how do these changes make themselves known in the realm of intimacy and relationships? For many, there is often a tangible impact on sexual performance, leading to a chain reaction of psychological effects such as anxiety or diminished confidence. This can be a delicate subject to approach with a partner, yet acknowledging these changes is vital. Rather than viewing them as a decline, they can be reframed as a call for a deeper understanding and connection.

Moreover, hormonal changes are influenced not solely by the passage of time but by lifestyle factors and overall health. Obesity, sedentary lifestyles, and chronic illnesses such as diabetes and cardiovascular disease can exacerbate the decline in testosterone levels. Therefore, adopting healthy lifestyle habits becomes paramount—not just as a means to maintain hormone levels, but to augment overall well-being and sexual health.

It's worth noting that hormonal changes don't spell the end of sexual intimacy. On the contrary, many men report rewarding sexual experiences well into their later years; they simply might require adjustments and adaptability to changing capacities. The focus might shift from quantity to quality, emphasising emotional intimacy and exploring new avenues of pleasure.

For those seeking solutions, a discussion with a healthcare provider can offer insights into potential treatments, such as testosterone replacement therapy (TRT). While TRT can be beneficial for some, it's not without risks and should be considered carefully and on an individual basis. Understanding the balance and timing of these therapies can be pivotal, as can recognising when lifestyle changes alone might suffice.

Inviting your partner into this conversation can bridge gaps in understanding and strengthen bonds. Openness about one's struggles and adaptations in the face of hormonal shifts can lead to shared resolutions. Together, couples can explore tactics to address these changes—whether through therapy, lifestyle adjustments, or simply fostering emotional closeness.

As we navigate these transitions, the narrative surrounding ageing and hormonal changes requires a shift. By focusing on growth, adaptation, and resilience, we can transform potential obstacles into opportunities for deeper connections. This phase of life, rather than a decline, can become a vivid new chapter where intimacy evolves into something even more profound. Embrace the shifts with curiosity and a willingness to adapt, knowing that each step is a testament to the remarkable tapestry of human experience.

# Chapter 4:
# Psychological Contributors
# to Libido Loss

Amidst the puzzle of understanding libido loss in men, psychological factors often play a pivotal role that can't be overlooked. Stress, for instance, has a stealthy way of infiltrating the mind, clouding desire and distancing one from intimate connections. The weight of depression and anxiety also bears down, cloaking the psyche in shadows that dim not only mood but the spark of attraction. It's a complex interplay, where one's emotional and mental well-being significantly influences sexual vitality. Recognising these contributors is the first step towards reclaiming that lost passion. Once identified, strategies such as cognitive-behavioural techniques and mindfulness practices can serve as powerful allies in the battle against libido diminution. The road to recovery invites an exploration of deeper self-awareness and conscious nurturing of mental health, empowering men to rediscover their passion and deepen their connections with their partners.

## Stress and Its Effect

Stress has a sneaky way of creeping into every aspect of life, and its impact on libido is often underestimated. In our fast-paced world, stress seems to be a constant companion, wreaking havoc on both mental and physical health. It's not just the big life events that pile on the pressure; even the daily grind can take a toll. Juggling work commitments, personal responsibilities, and social obligations leaves little room for relaxation, and before you know it, stress is knocking on the door of your bedroom, uninvited and unwanted.

The link between stress and libido is rooted in our body's physiological response. When stress levels rise, the body reacts with a "fight or flight" response, releasing hormones like cortisol and adrenaline. This response, although crucial for survival in dangerous situations, can become detrimental when constantly activated. High levels of cortisol can disrupt the balance of sex hormones, leading to a decrease in desire. Moreover, the physical symptoms of stress, such as muscle tension and fatigue, can make the act of intimacy feel more like a chore than a pleasure.

This hormonal upheaval doesn't work in isolation; it intertwines with psychological factors, creating a complex web that can be hard to untangle. Stress can lead to feelings of anxiety and depression, both of which are known libido dampeners. The mind becomes preoccupied with worries and anxieties, making it difficult to focus on intimacy. In turn, the lack of desire can become a source of stress itself, creating a vicious cycle that's tough to break.

Perhaps the most insidious effect of stress is how it affects self-esteem. When stress leads to burnout, it can alter one's self-perception, causing a man to feel less attractive or capable. This negative self-image can further compound feelings of inadequacy, making it difficult to engage with a partner intimately. The inner dialogue becomes a relentless critic, undermining confidence and suppressing sexual appetite.

Fortunately, understanding stress and its effects paves the way for effective strategies to combat it. The first step is recognising the various sources of stress in one's life. This awareness allows for the implementation of stress management techniques, such as mindfulness, meditation, or even simple deep-breathing exercises.

Taking time to disconnect from the hustle and bustle and focus on relaxation can significantly reduce stress levels, bringing a sense of calm back into one's life.

Open communication with a partner also plays a crucial role in mitigating stress. Sharing burdens and discussing feelings alleviates the pressure of facing challenges alone. This kind of emotional support strengthens the relationship and fosters an environment in which sexual desire can flourish once again. Empathy and understanding cultivate closeness, which is often more powerful than any external remedy.

Another vital aspect lies in setting realistic expectations for oneself and one's partner. Life's demands are ever-present, yet expecting to maintain a perfect balance is unrealistic and can lead to disappointment. Embracing imperfections and prioritising self-care over perfectionism can ease stress levels, naturally rejuvenating libido.

Moreover, integrating physical activity into one's routine serves as an effective stress buster. Exercise releases endorphins, the body's natural mood elevators, and helps regulate hormone levels. Whether it's a brisk walk, a session at the gym, or practising yoga, regular physical activity can make a world of difference in how stress is managed and how libido responds.

Lastly, when stress seems overwhelming, seeking professional guidance can provide the tools needed to handle life's hurdles effectively. Therapy or counselling offers a safe space to explore stress triggers and develop coping mechanisms that are tailored to individual needs. Don't hesitate to reach out for help; it's a courageous step towards regaining control.

In conclusion, while stress is an inevitable part of life, its effects on libido need not be permanent. By understanding the interplay between stress and sexual desire, men can break free from the cycle and pave the way towards a more fulfilling intimate life. With the right approach, stress can be managed and passion reignited, strengthening both the individual and their relationship.

## Depression and Anxiety

In the intricate dance of mental health, depression and anxiety often lead, casting shadows that extend far beyond the realm of mood and emotion. Among their impacts is a notable decline in libido, a deeply personal and often distressing shift for men and their partners. Understanding how these conditions can affect sexual desire requires looking at the complex interplay between mental health and sexual functioning.

Depression, often characterised by pervasive sadness and a lack of interest or pleasure in activities, can significantly dampen sexual desire. It's more than just feeling emotionally low; depression affects neurotransmitters in the brain that are crucial for regulating mood and sexual arousal. The production of dopamine, which plays a key role in the sensation of pleasure and reward, is often disrupted, leading to diminished libido. In this context, a decline in sexual interest is not merely a symptom but a reflection of a more extensive emotional disconnection.

Anxiety, which frequently coexists with depression, compounds these challenges. Often described as a persistent state of unease or worry, anxiety can create a cycle of fear and stress that impairs sexual performance and enjoyment. The body's fight-or-flight response, a hallmark of anxiety, hijacks the nervous system, redirecting energy away from non-essential functions like sexual response. This physiological shift often results in struggles with arousal and performance, further entrenching anxiety's grip on libido.

For many men, admitting to experiencing these mental health challenges can be fraught with difficulty. Society's often unrealistic expectations of stoicism and resilience can discourage open discussion about feelings of depression and anxiety, especially when they seem to affect one's libido—a deeply personal aspect of masculinity and intimacy. Breaking through these barriers requires acknowledging that experiencing such mental health difficulty doesn't diminish a man's strength or capability.

One powerful approach to addressing libido loss linked to depression and anxiety is recognising the need for professional support. Therapeutic interventions, such as cognitive-behavioural therapy (CBT), have proven effective in addressing the distorted thinking patterns and behavioural responses that fuel both depression and anxiety. These therapies empower individuals to navigate their mental health challenges actively, fostering strategies to alleviate symptoms and improving overall wellbeing.

Meanwhile, medication can also play a part in the broader management of these mental health conditions. Antidepressant and anti-anxiety medications, while potentially beneficial, may have mixed effects on libido. Some medications can inadvertently dampen sexual desire further, which implies the necessity for ongoing communication with healthcare providers to tailor treatment plans that consider not just mental health outcomes but sexual health as well.

While professional help is indispensable, cultivating a supportive environment at home can work wonders alongside professional treatment. Honest communication with a partner about the experiences of depression and anxiety can open avenues to shared understanding and shared problem-solving. Empathy from a partner can transform what feels like an isolating struggle into a journey towards recovery supported by teamwork and mutual affection.

Furthermore, lifestyle modifications can offer complementary benefits. Regular physical activity, a balanced diet, and adequate sleep are well-documented contributors to enhanced mood and reduced anxiety. Exercise, in particular, has the dual benefit of enhancing physical health and boosting mental fortitude due to the release of endorphins, which are natural mood lifters. Such lifestyle improvements, although part of a broader chapter in this book, can specifically underpin mental wellbeing and, by extension, bolster sexual health.

It's crucial not to overlook the role of self-compassion in this equation. Men struggling with libido loss due to depression or anxiety often wrestle with self-criticism and shame, feelings that can further entrench low self-worth and depressive symptoms. Practising self-kindness and patience can counteract these negative tendencies, paving the way for more positive self-perception and, ultimately, a healthier relationship with one's own sexuality.

This journey through depression and anxiety towards restored libido is not linear, nor is it without its challenges. However, armed with understanding, empathy, and practical strategies, it's possible to navigate these mental health hurdles effectively. Emphasising progress over perfection, and recognising the small victories along the way, can profoundly impact one's journey towards renewed intimacy and connection.

Depression and anxiety do not have to be the enduring villains of sexuality and romantic relationships. Rather, they can be seen as challenges to be understood and mastered, with the potential to deepen personal insight and emotional resilience. By embracing comprehensive approaches that include professional help, lifestyle changes, and empathy both for oneself and from partners, the pathway towards overcoming libido loss and restoring passionate intimacy is decidedly achievable.

## Mental Health Strategies

Understanding the intricate relationship between mental well-being and libido is fundamental for men experiencing a drop in sexual desire. This section delves into effective strategies to manage mental health, offering a pathway to rejuvenate one's sexual drive. A decrease in libido often goes hand-in-hand with stress, depression, or anxiety, which means tackling these issues can be pivotal in restoring not just sexual desire but overall quality of life.

First and foremost, the importance of acknowledging one's mental state cannot be overstated. It might seem daunting to introspect and identify issues like stress or anxiety. However, self-awareness is a practical starting point. You must give yourself permission to admit that mental health factors are intertwined with libido fluctuations. Recognising this is not a sign of weakness; it's a critical step towards empowerment and control over your sexual health.

Developing effective coping mechanisms is crucial. Mindfulness practices such as meditation and breathing exercises can significantly alleviate symptoms of stress and anxiety. These techniques don't require complex tools or extensive time commitments. Even a few minutes daily can improve your mental clarity and relaxation. As you ease the mind, you create a favourable environment for libido to thrive naturally.

Exercise serves as another vital mental health strategy. Physical activity is not just beneficial for physical health; it has profound effects on mental well-being too. Engaging in regular exercise releases endorphins, which are natural mood lifters. By incorporating fitness routines into your lifestyle, you may find yourself more resilient against daily stressors, aiding in mental balance and an increase in sexual drive.

You can't overlook the power of social support. Successful management of mental health often involves strong connections with friends, family, or partners. Sharing your experiences with trusted individuals offers emotional relief and prevents any feeling of isolation. A conversation over coffee or a heartfelt discussion with your partner might open up new avenues for understanding and mutual support, enhancing emotional closeness and eventually reigniting libido.

Cognitive Behavioural Therapy (CBT) can also be a game-changer for men battling low mood and anxiety affecting their libido. CBT helps restructure harmful thought patterns and develop healthier perspectives. Access to this kind of therapy is essential for those eager to tackle psychological barriers head-on. A trained therapist can guide you through specific exercises to reframe anxious or depressive thoughts, unlocking pathways to enhanced sexual desire.

It's worth considering the role of professional counselling, especially if you're struggling to manage mental health on your own. Counsellors specialise in offering insight and strategies tailored to individual needs. They provide a safe environment to explore underlying issues, allowing you to address them with confidence and direction. Such professional guidance can be transformative, as it empowers you to rediscover your passion and sexual vitality.

Mindful journaling is another method to enhance mental well-being. By recording thoughts and feelings regularly, you get a clearer picture of what's influencing your mental and sexual health. Journaling helps you track patterns and triggers, and it's a private avenue for expression. This practice can lead to self-discovery and personal growth, indirectly boosting your libido as you become more attuned to your internal workings.

Dietary choices may also influence mental health in ways that affect libido. Certain nutrients support brain health, indirectly sustaining a more robust sexual drive. Omega-3 fatty acids, found in fish like salmon, and vitamins B and D play essential roles in mood regulation. Maintaining a balanced diet rich in these nutrients can bolster mental wellness, creating conditions conducive to a healthy libido.

Improving sleep hygiene is an often overlooked yet effective strategy. Poor sleep can exacerbate mental health conditions like anxiety and depression, thereby diminishing sexual desire. Ensuring that you have consistent, high-quality sleep can significantly enhance mood and energy levels. Establishing a bedtime routine and creating a restful sleeping environment can help you achieve the restorative rest your body needs.

Lastly, practising gratitude can shift focus from stressors to positive aspects of life, enhancing mental health and, consequently, libido. Regularly acknowledging things you are thankful for, whether it's your health, relationships, or achievements, contributes to an optimistic outlook. An improved mood and mental outlook can naturally uplift your sexual desire as you view intimacy from a place of abundance rather than deficit.

The journey towards overcoming libido loss through mental health strategies is about taking proactive steps and making conscious decisions to bolster emotional and psychological well-being. These approaches, when applied consistently, have the potential to revitalize not only your mental state but also your intimate life, paving the way for renewed passion and fulfilment in your relationship.

# Chapter 5:
# Physical Health and Its
# Impact on Libido

Physical health isn't just about being active or eating well—it's a cornerstone for maintaining a vibrant libido. When the body thrives, so does our sexual desire. Lifestyle choices like regular exercise can enhance blood flow and boost mood, creating a positive feedback loop for libido. Conversely, chronic health conditions such as diabetes or cardiovascular diseases can impede sexual function, revealing how intricately linked physical well-being is with sexual vitality. Embracing a balanced lifestyle not only fortifies the body but also supports a fulfilling intimate life. By making health a priority, you're not just enhancing overall well-being; you're laying the groundwork for reigniting passion and closeness in your relationships. Understand that the path to revitalised intimacy begins with taking care of the physical self, a commitment that yields benefits far beyond the bedroom.

## The Link with Lifestyle Choices

A thriving lifestyle is often the bedrock of robust physical health, and its influence on libido is profound. Men struggling with a decline in sexual desire may find the answer lies less in a medical condition and more in the lifestyle choices quietly shaping their lives. This isn't merely about avoiding bad habits; it's about embracing choices that support and enhance sexual vitality. Small changes, over time, can accumulate into significant improvements, offering not just hope but tangible results.

Diet is a cornerstone of these lifestyle choices. What you put on your plate can impact hormonal balance, cardiovascular health, and energy levels—all vital components of maintaining a healthy libido. Prioritising whole, unprocessed foods rich in nutrients fuels the body and supports peak performance in all aspects of life, including the bedroom. An indulgence in sugar-laden foods, highly processed meals, and excessive dairy can dampen libido by contributing to poor blood flow and altered hormone levels. Such dietary habits are like unseen thieves stealing away your vigour.

But let's be clear: not all consequences of dietary choices are negative. The Mediterranean diet, for example, is renowned for its beneficial effects. Packed with fruits, vegetables, healthy fats, and lean proteins, this diet supports heart health, which is intimately connected to sexual performance. A healthy heart pumps blood efficiently, ensuring that sexual organs receive the oxygen and nutrients they need to function optimally. Incorporating these kinds of dietary patterns isn't just about seeing immediate results—it's about establishing a sustainable lifestyle that continues to nourish desire.

Beyond food, physical activity plays a critical role in enhancing libido. Regular exercise boosts cardiovascular health, fosters hormonal balance, and reduces stress—all factors contributing to increased sexual desire. An active lifestyle ensures that energy levels remain high, blood circulation improves, and confidence gets a boost with each achieved fitness milestone. Practices like strength training, yoga, or even a brisk daily walk can have a transformational effect. They're not merely tasks to check off a list; they can become a satisfying part of daily life, making exercise less of a chore and more of a joy.

Moreover, exercise triggers the release of endorphins—nature's own pleasure chemicals—which not only improve mood but also increase feelings of pleasure and satisfaction. This chemical cocktail effectively fights off stress and anxiety, common psychological barriers to libido. When engaging in regular physical activity, you're not just training your body but also nurturing mental health, creating a virtuous cycle that feeds into better sexual health.

Sleep—often the most overlooked aspect of lifestyle—is paramount in maintaining a healthy libido. Chronic sleep deprivation can lead to reduced testosterone levels, increased stress hormones, and overall fatigue, all of which constrict sexual desire. Conversely, good quality sleep improves mental health, hormone balance, and energy reserve. Therefore, establishing healthy sleep routines isn't just for rest's sake; it's integral to maintaining a fulfilling sexual life. It could be as simple as following a consistent sleep schedule or creating a bedroom environment conducive to rest.

Alcohol and substance use are factors that need careful consideration. While a glass of wine might feel like it sets the mood for romance, habitual or excessive consumption can have the opposite effect, leading to decreased libido and sexual performance. Alcohol, particularly, can suppress testosterone production and inhibit the central nervous system's responsiveness, dampening both arousal and satisfaction. Moderation is key, and recognising the fine balance between occasional indulgence and routine use can safeguard your sexual health.

We've barely scratched the surface of how these choices impact libido, but their influence is unmistakable. Engaging in a lifestyle health check—a thoughtful analysis of your diet, exercise, sleep, and substance use—can offer crucial insights into the potential triggers of libido decline. From there, an actionable plan to introduce healthier habits can be crafted, turning potential pitfalls into stepping stones toward enhanced sexual vitality.

However, it's important to acknowledge the interconnectivity of lifestyle choices. Making changes in one area often has a cascading effect on others. Improving diet, for instance, often leads to increased energy and motivation for regular exercise. Better physical activity levels can improve sleep, and a well-rested body is less likely to crave unhealthy foods or alcohol. Understanding this ripple effect is crucial in optimising lifestyle changes for maximum benefit to your sexual health.

Finally, the journey to improving sexual desire through lifestyle changes doesn't have to be undertaken alone. Involve your partner in these changes for mutual support and understanding. Sharing activities like cooking healthy meals together or embarking on a fitness journey can be bonding experiences, reinforcing emotional and physical closeness. This partnership not only aids in sustaining lifestyle changes but also enhances relationship dynamics, creating a more fulfilling and intimate connection.

Remember, true change is about cultivating habits that harmonise with your personal desires and daily life, not imposing unrealistic standards. It's about small, consistent steps towards a lifestyle that supports not just your libido but your overall well-being. As these changes accumulate, the results will speak for themselves, manifesting in renewed energy, passion, and a newfound confidence in your intimate relationships.

## Chronic Health Conditions

Chronic health conditions are like the relentless companions that walk a parallel path alongside many men as they navigate their lives. These conditions, existing long before libido loss knocks at the door, can insidiously impact a man's sexual desire and performance. Understanding the intersection between chronic health issues and libido is essential, not only for managing symptoms but also for fostering intimate and fulfilling relationships.

One of the most significant chronic ailments with known repercussions on libido is diabetes. This condition affects millions of men worldwide and brings about a cascade of changes in the body, including nerve damage and reduced blood flow. Both are significant factors in erectile dysfunction, which can then lead to a decrease in libido as a result. The strain of managing diabetes, coupled with its physiological challenges, can result in a steeper decline in sexual interest and activity.

Cardiovascular disease is another prevalent condition with a notable impact on sexual health. It's more than just the heart that's affected; the circulation system plays a pivotal role in maintaining sexual function. When arteries clog and blood flow is restricted, it doesn't just affect energy levels—it hits home in the bedroom, too. As sexual arousal relies heavily on blood flow, any impediment can diminish this essential bodily function, often leading to frustration and a sense of failure.

Then there's hypertension, or high blood pressure, a silent condition that can sneak up on men and chip away at their libido. Medications used to treat hypertension, such as beta-blockers, have been documented to further suppress sexual desire, adding yet another layer of complexity. This creates a vicious cycle where one's efforts to manage blood pressure inadvertently compromise sexual health, leaving many men in a bind between necessary medical treatment and personal fulfillment.

Chronic pain conditions, such as arthritis or fibromyalgia, also exert a powerful influence on libido. These ailments, characterised by persistent pain and fatigue, can make the thought of sexual activity exhausting at best and impossible at worst. When pain becomes a central focus, the mental and physical energy required to maintain sexual desire is severely taxed, often leaving intimacy on the backburner.

Beyond physical symptoms, the emotional toll of chronic illness cannot be overlooked. The stress of constant pain management, appointments, and daily limitations can lead to a significant emotional burden, impacting mental health and sexual wellbeing. Depression and anxiety are common companions of chronic conditions, amplifying feelings of isolation and reducing sexual interest as a result. These emotional challenges add yet another layer of complexity to an already intricate situation.

Some conditions, like obesity, are both a chronic health issue and a significant factor influencing libido. Obesity can lead to hormonal changes, reducing testosterone levels which are crucial for maintaining sexual desire. It can also impact self-esteem and body image, which play critical roles in sexual confidence and attraction. The weight of these challenges can be both literal and metaphorical, affecting every facet of sexual health and wellbeing.

Respiratory conditions, such as chronic obstructive pulmonary disease (COPD), can also undermine libido, primarily due to physical fatigue and decreased stamina. When breathing becomes laboured, energy levels are sapped, leaving little reserve for sexual activity. This physical limitation can create barriers to not only desire but also the ability to engage in intimate moments comfortably.

Given the multifaceted nature of chronic health conditions, a tailored and compassionate approach is necessary to manage their impact on libido. It's crucial to foster open communication about these challenges within relationships. Discussing health concerns and their effects candidly with a partner can forge a sense of understanding and collaboration, crucial elements for navigating the rough waters of intimacy diminished by chronic illness.

Moreover, addressing chronic health conditions often requires a comprehensive approach involving healthcare professionals. Working alongside medical providers ensures therapies align with an individual's sexual health objectives, minimising medication side effects and exploring alternative treatment options when possible. This collaborative care can help strike a balance between maintaining overall health and nurturing sexual desire.

Efforts to mitigate the impact of chronic conditions should also focus on lifestyle modifications. Prioritising a balanced diet, regular exercise, and adequate sleep serves to bolster overall health and can lead to improvements in libido. Lifestyle choices hold remarkable potential in managing both chronic conditions and their downstream effects on sexual wellbeing.

In this journey, patience and persistence become invaluable allies. While chronic conditions might initially appear as immovable barriers, small, consistent changes can lead to significant improvements in the long run. For men grappling with these challenges, understanding is key—it's not just about managing a condition but reshaping one's life and relationship with their own body.

Ultimately, the marriage of chronic health management and intimacy requires adaptability, resilience, and an openness to new strategies. By embracing these qualities, men and their partners can forge paths through the challenges posed by chronic conditions and find ways to foster a renewed physical and emotional connection. The journey may be complex, but with knowledge, support, and perseverance, it is one that can be navigated successfully.

## Exercise and its Benefits

Good health and an active lifestyle are tightly interwoven, and exercise plays a significant role in this dynamic. For men experiencing a decline in libido, regular physical activity can be transformative, not only in terms of physical health but also for mental well-being. Developing a structured exercise regimen can reignite passion and intimacy by addressing some of the root causes of libido loss.

When you engage in physical activity, your body experiences a multitude of beneficial changes. Firstly, exercise enhances cardiovascular health, which is crucial for sexual function. A healthy heart can pump blood more efficiently, ensuring that all organs, including the sexual organs, receive adequate blood flow. This improved circulation directly impacts erectile function and overall sexual performance.

Additionally, regular exercise can lead to weight loss and muscle gain. Maintaining a healthy weight and increased muscle mass can boost testosterone levels, as excess body fat can lead to hormone imbalance. Increased testosterone can help rejuvenate sexual desire, providing a natural boost to libido. Remember that not every form of exercise suits everyone—finding what works best for you, whether it's resistance training, aerobic exercises, or flexibility workouts, is key to sustained engagement.

Exercise also has significant psychological benefits that can help tackle libido decline. Physical activity acts as a powerful stress reliever. It prompts the release of endorphins, those 'feel-good' chemicals that naturally boost your mood and reduce stress levels. Lower stress levels equate to higher chances of improved libido, as stress is a known factor in diminishing sexual desire and performance.

Mental health is greatly enhanced through regular exercise, assisting those dealing with depression and anxiety. Both conditions can severely impact one's sexual desire. A workout routine can improve sleep quality, lift mood, and increase energy levels, all contributing to a better outlook on life and improved sexual health.

Another key benefit of exercise is the enhancement of body image and self-esteem. Feeling good about your physical appearance can improve confidence in intimate settings. This confidence may, in turn, be attractive to your partner, fostering a more fulfilling relationship.

Yet the impact of exercise extends beyond individual benefits. Engaging in physical activities with your partner—like walking, dancing, or sports—can increase emotional bonds and improve communication. This shared experience can reignite passion and create a sense of teamwork in overcoming challenges associated with libido loss.

It's essential to integrate variety in your exercise routine to maintain interest and enthusiasm. Incorporating different activities not only keeps things exciting but also works out various muscle groups, ensuring a balanced improvement in fitness. Incorporate activities that are enjoyable and achievable to prevent burnout and ensure long-term commitment.

Of course, before beginning any new exercise regime, it would be wise to consult with a healthcare professional to tailor a program suited to your personal health requirements. Ensuring your routine aligns with your lifestyle and any pre-existing health conditions can optimise your outcomes and reduce the risk of injury.

In conclusion, exercise is a powerful, multifaceted solution for improving libido. Its physical benefits are matched by mental and emotional gains, making it a holistic approach to addressing sexual health. Remember, it's about adopting a mindset where small, consistent changes lead to sustainable results. Embracing physical activity not only transforms your health but can breathe new life into intimate relationships, helping you reconnect with yourself and your partner.

# Chapter 6:
# Relationship Dynamics

In navigating the intricate tapestry of **relationship dynamics**, it's vital to understand that building robust connections goes beyond mere physical attraction; it requires a deep commitment to *effective communication* and emotional closeness. This realm is where couples find harmony by engaging in open dialogues, embracing vulnerability, and actively resolving conflicts. By fostering an environment where honesty is prioritised, trust can flourish, enabling both partners to venture into joint explorations of solutions, especially pertinent when libido wanes. As you strengthen these bonds, remember that your relationship's resilience often mirrors your capacity to adapt and mutually support one another. These dynamics aren't static; they ebb and flow, demanding continuous attention and effort. Yet with patience and understanding, you can transform challenges into opportunities for growth, paving the path toward rejuvenated intimacy.

## Communication with Your Partner

Effective communication is the bedrock of any healthy relationship. It becomes even more critical when facing the sensitive issue of declining libido. Addressing sexual desire involves vulnerable conversations, necessitating openness and honesty from both partners. When actually engaging in these discussions, remember: it's not just about talking, but really listening and understanding.

Begin by establishing an environment where both you and your partner feel safe to express feelings and concerns. You might think about a neutral setting, perhaps away from the bedroom, to start the dialogue. Approach these talks with empathy and patience, acknowledging that this isn't merely a physical concern but one that intertwines with emotion and self-worth. By building a foundation of trust, you lay the groundwork for genuine exploration of the issues at hand.

It's essential to approach these conversations without fault or blame. A decline in libido can stem from a multitude of factors, and it's rarely a result of just one person's actions or characteristics. Use "I" statements to express how you're feeling. For instance, "I feel anxious about our intimacy" is much less accusatory than "You never want to be intimate anymore." This distinction can significantly shift the tone of the conversation, making it constructive rather than confrontational.

Vulnerability is pivotal. Sharing your fears and insecurities about your libido, and encouraging your partner to share theirs, opens the door to deeper emotional closeness. When partners allow themselves to be vulnerable, it can strengthen their bond and foster a deeper understanding of each other. However, being vulnerable is often easier said than done. It requires courage and a commitment to working through discomfort. This kind of emotional exposure can sometimes feel daunting, but the rewards—empathy, support, and eventual growth—are well worth the effort.

Don't underestimate the power of setting aside regular times to check in with one another. Whether it's a weekly or monthly practice, having a routine for open discussion can alleviate lingering tensions or unspoken worries before they snowball into larger issues. This kind of structure not only facilitates ongoing communication but also demonstrates a commitment to working together on the issues at hand.

It's equally important to establish a tone of mutual support. When discussing changes in sexual desire, listen actively to your partner's concerns without interrupting. Show empathy by reflecting on their feelings: "It seems like you're feeling..." is a powerful phrase to use. This not only validates their emotions but also promotes a deeper understanding between you both. By feeling heard, partners are more likely to feel secure in expressing their full range of emotions and thoughts, paving the way for more productive discussions.

Non-verbal communication is just as crucial. Eye contact, touch, and facial expressions convey understanding and empathy. A gentle touch on the arm or a sincere gaze can speak volumes, reinforcing verbal affirmations. These non-verbal cues help to maintain a connection even when words become complex or emotionally charged.

It's natural to encounter emotional turbulence during these dialogues. Some conversations may bring up past hurts or misunderstandings. In such moments, practise patience and propose a break if things become overwhelming. Agree on a time to resume the conversation once emotions have settled. This prevents heightened emotions from dictating the discussion and gives both partners time to reflect on what's been said.

Complete ownership and responsibility are key components of these dialogues. If your libido issues stem from personal or lifestyle choices, acknowledge them openly. Admitting, "I haven't been taking care of my health as I should," invites a collaborative problem-solving approach, rather than defensiveness. On the flip side, if your partner is struggling with something unrelated that affects your intimacy, encourage them to explore these factors openly. Compassion lies in the willingness to tackle these issues together.

Problem-solving together is a natural progression of effective communication. Brainstorm solutions that both of you are comfortable with and consider seeking professional guidance if needed. Consulting a therapist or counselor who specialises in sexual health can provide additional strategies and insights, fostering an environment where both partners feel empowered and understood.

Recognise that these dialogues are iterative rather than one-off events. Expect setbacks and celebrate small victories along the way. Each conversation should be viewed as a stepping stone towards a healthier and more fulfilling relationship.

Finally, maintaining a sense of humour can be incredibly beneficial. While libido discussions are undeniably serious, finding small moments of light-heartedness or shared laughter can diffuse tension. Humour can bridge gaps in understanding and remind you both of the love that underpins your journey together.

The aim is to journey through these conversations not as opponents, but as allies. Openness, understanding, and patience are the guiding lights that will illuminate the path through challenges. With each step, you'll not only be working through current issues but also fortifying the overall resilience and depth of your relationship. In the end, the goal isn't just to resolve an issue but to redefine what intimacy means in your partnership, allowing both liberty and intimacy to thrive side by side.

## Emotional Closeness and Conflict

In navigating the complexities of emotional closeness and conflict within relationships, particularly when addressing challenges related to declining sexual desire, it becomes essential to consider both the emotional and psychological landscapes. At its core, emotional closeness is the foundation upon which intimacy is built. However, when this closeness is strained or challenged, conflict often finds fertile ground. Addressing this knotty issue begins with understanding how emotional connection or its absence can manifest in accompanied differences, disagreements, and potentially discord.

Conflict in relationships can come from many sources—unmet expectations, miscommunication, or the feeling of being misunderstood. Yet, at the heart of these issues often lies a fundamental need for emotional connection. When sexual desire in men wanes, it might be tempting to focus solely on physical or hormonal causes. However, the emotional aspect shouldn't be underestimated. For many men, emotional intimacy can be deeply tied to their experience of sexual connection. Therefore, when conflict arises, it may sometimes act as a mask for underlying emotional wounds or needs that haven't been addressed.

Developing emotional closeness involves a kind of vulnerable openness that many find challenging to achieve. It requires not just talking but sharing—a willingness to express one's fears, hopes, and experiences without fear of judgement. This depth of sharing can help partners understand each other beyond the conflicts at hand, fostering a deeper emotional bond. When emotional closeness flourishes, it often creates a buffer against misunderstandings and can make resolving conflicts more straightforward.

However, this isn't to say that achieving emotional closeness is without its hurdles. Some men may find it difficult to articulate their emotions, especially when societal norms or personal upbringing have taught them to view such expressions as a sign of weakness. This reticence can lead to feelings of isolation or inadequacy, exacerbating conflicts rather than resolving them. Encouraging open dialogue within a relationship by creating a safe and supportive environment is crucial.

Strategies for enhancing emotional closeness and reducing conflict should always consider both partners' desires and comfort zones. Finding common ground through shared experiences like new activities or revisiting forgotten hobbies can serve as a powerful emotional connector. These shared moments can rekindle not just affection but kindle a genuine interest in each other's evolving identities and needs.

Additionally, empathy plays a substantial role in diffusing conflict and building closeness. By placing oneself in the partner's shoes, individuals can better understand their partner's perspectives, acknowledging that each person experiences the relationship uniquely. Such understanding promotes patience and forbearance during challenging times, allowing conflicts to become opportunities for growth rather than stumbling blocks.

Regular, intentional communication also stands as a pillar in maintaining emotional closeness. Setting aside dedicated time to connect and discuss each other's lives, aspirations, and challenges ensures both partners feel valued and understood. It's equally important to celebrate successes and transformations, no matter how small, as this reinforces positive emotional connections.

Sometimes, the journey to enhanced emotional closeness and reduced conflict may necessitate external guidance. Couples counselling can provide valuable insights and tools to navigate the complexities that might be challenging for partners to deal with independently. Experienced therapists can offer a neutral perspective and equip partners with communication skills essential for resolving deeper issues.

It's worth noting that no relationship is devoid of conflict. When handled constructively, conflict isn't a sign of failure—but rather a chance to strengthen the emotional fabric of a partnership. By learning to resolve conflicts healthily, couples can prevent the unfortunate cycle of blame and resentment that can distance partners emotionally.

Ultimately, emotional closeness and conflict go hand in hand in this intricate dance we call relationships. For men facing the decline of sexual desire, addressing the emotional components is just as vital as tackling any physical or psychological factors. Embracing emotional vulnerability, fostering genuine connections, and navigating conflicts with empathy and resilience are indispensable steps on this journey towards revitalised intimacy and lasting relationships.

## Joint Exploration of Solutions

When it comes to navigating the complexities of dwindling libido, a joint exploration of solutions often serves as a cornerstone for rejuvenating relationships. At the heart of this venture lies the commitment to fostering a partnership where both individuals can openly communicate their desires, concerns, and aspirations. This isn't just about tackling an issue in isolation; it's about embarking on a shared journey to rediscover intimacy and connection. To undertake this journey, both partners must engage in an active dialogue, drawing on empathy and understanding. A relationship thrives when there's a mutual investment in finding sustainable solutions. Such an endeavour often requires stepping outside of one's comfort zone to embrace the vulnerability that accompanies true intimacy.

One of the initial steps in this collaborative exploration is setting the stage for open communication. Designating time and space for candid discussions can be transformative. It's crucial to ensure these conversations are free from distractions, allowing both partners to be fully present. Effective communication doesn't just involve expressing one's needs; it also demands active listening. Each partner should feel seen, heard, and valued. Through these dialogues, couples can gain insights into the underlying factors impacting libido and work together to address them. It's about cultivating an atmosphere where each partner feels safe to share their struggles and triumphs without fear of judgment or reproach.

In many cases, joint exploration will reveal that simple changes in daily routines can have profound impacts. For instance, couples might decide to incorporate regular "relationship check-ins" to assess how they are both feeling. This is akin to taking the temperature of the relationship, identifying areas that require attention before they escalate into larger issues. By regularly engaging in these assessments, couples maintain an ongoing conversation about their emotional and physical needs—an integral step in rekindling desire.

Physical activity can also serve as a bonding experience, and leveraging its benefits is another avenue that couples can explore together. Whether it's committing to a daily walk, practising yoga, or even dancing in the living room, shared physical activities can enhance both emotional closeness and physical health. Exercise naturally boosts endorphins, reducing stress levels and potentially increasing sexual desire. By prioritising activities they both enjoy, couples can cultivate a sense of teamwork while also addressing a key contributor to libido loss.

Couples might also explore the pivotal role that lifestyle adjustments can play in this journey. Understanding that nutrition, sleep, and even media consumption can significantly impact one's libido, they might opt to curate a joint plan that encourages healthier habits. Setting goals related to diet, sleep hygiene, and digital detoxing can be both empowering and unifying. For example, cooking meals together not only ensures healthier eating but also introduces moments of connection and collaboration. Emphasising sleep quality and practising good hygiene can lead to improved mood and energy levels—key components of sexual desire.

Moreover, part of this collaborative effort involves educating themselves about various therapeutic approaches. While therapy and counselling are traditionally viewed as individual or private pursuits, joint sessions can yield substantial benefits. Couples' counselling provides a platform to explore emotional patterns and joint dynamics that may have gone unnoticed. Through therapy, couples can learn strategies to better manage stress and mental health issues—often significant barriers to maintaining libido. Furthermore, therapists can guide couples in redefining their understanding of intimacy, moving beyond mere physical encounters to a more holistic connection.

However, a successful joint exploration also requires an openness to redefining roles and expectations within the relationship. It's common to fall into patterns where expectations are shaped by past experiences or societal norms. By consciously choosing to challenge and redefine these roles, couples can foster a more authentic partnership. This might involve a role reversal in household responsibilities or challenging gender-based assumptions around libido. Such transformations can create a more balanced dynamic, allowing both partners to feel more fulfilled and less burdened, which can naturally enhance sexual desire.

Furthermore, this journey is enhanced by recognising and celebrating small victories. Success in addressing libido issues often comes incrementally rather than through dramatic changes. By acknowledging and celebrating these steps, whether it's increased closeness or improved communication, couples reinforce their shared commitment. This celebration doesn't have to be grand; sometimes, a simple acknowledgment or a thank-you note is enough to strengthen the bond.

Ultimately, exploring solutions together isn't just about reigniting passion; it's about building a resilient, adaptable relationship that can weather future challenges. It requires effort and dedication from both partners, but the rewards are extensive. As couples navigate this pathway, they'll likely discover new forms of closeness and intimacy that enrich their partnership beyond the confines of sexual desire. This endeavour, when approached with patience and compassion, can transform not just their sexual relationship but also the very fabric of their lives together.

# Chapter 7:
## Addressing Lifestyle Factors

Our daily habits hold the key to unlocking renewed sexual vitality. When we prioritise balanced nutrition, rejuvenating sleep, and mindful moderation of substances, we're not just ticking health boxes but crafting a fertile ground for desire and connection. Consider how the vibrant colours of fruits and vegetables signal a promise of vitality, or how restful sleep rejuvenates both body and mind, fostering the clarity and energy needed for intimacy. Meanwhile, recognising the thin line between substance use and misuse allows us to make conscious choices that preserve our well-being. By nurturing these lifestyle pillars, we create a ripple effect that extends beyond our own libido, enriching relationships and cultivating a life infused with passion and purpose. It's a commitment to a lifestyle that celebrates health as its own form of intimacy, leading to more profound connections and a revitalised sense of self.

## The Importance of Nutrition

Understanding the connection between nutrition and libido is vital when addressing lifestyle factors that influence sexual desire. Nutrition plays a pivotal role in overall health, particularly in regulating the systems that govern sexual health. The body's nutritional needs are closely linked with its hormonal balance, energy levels, and physical wellbeing. All these factors contribute significantly to maintaining a healthy libido.

Poor dietary choices can lead to a plethora of health issues that ultimately affect sexual desire, ranging from weight gain to chronic illnesses. An excessive intake of processed foods, saturated fats, and sugars can diminish vitality and reduce hormonal balance, which is crucial for having a healthy libido. Conversely, a well-balanced diet rich in essential nutrients provides the foundation for enhanced sexual health. Whole foods like fruits, vegetables, lean proteins, and healthy fats should be included to ensure that the body gets what it needs to support sexual function effectively.

Fruits and vegetables can't be overlooked in this discussion. They are replete with antioxidants, vitamins, and minerals that boost circulation and heart health, two critical factors for productive sexual performance. For instance, foods high in antioxidants help ward off inflammation and reduce oxidative stress, which can otherwise negatively impact sexual health. Moreover, enhanced blood circulation means better stamina and responsiveness, directly impacting one's libido.

Proteins, especially lean sources such as fish, chicken, and legumes, play a crucial role as well. These foods provide amino acids necessary for the production of neurotransmitters, like dopamine and serotonin, chemicals directly related to pleasure and reward pathways in the brain. Adequate protein intake can improve mood, boost energy levels, and thus indirectly enhance libido. Importantly, omega-3 fatty acids in fish are known to improve heart health and endothelial function, both of which are imperative for a healthy sex life.

Besides vegetables and proteins, whole grains and healthy fats must be part of a balanced nutrition plan. Whole grains provide essential fibre, which helps maintain steady blood sugar levels, a crucial factor in regulating mood and energy. This stability can lead to more consistent energy levels and a healthier libido. Additionally, healthy fats, such as those found in avocados, nuts, and olive oil, support hormonal health.

Fats are necessary for the production of hormones like testosterone, which are crucial for sexual arousal and libido.

Hydration is another essential factor often overlooked in discussions about nutrition and libido. Water intake influences nearly every metabolic process in the body. Dehydration can lead to fatigue, headaches, and concentration difficulties, indirectly affecting sexual interest. Maintaining proper hydration ensures that the body functions optimally, facilitating better energy levels and overall resilience.

Moreover, the implications of nutrition on mental health can't be dismissed. A nutritious diet supports cognitive health, which is vital when managing psychological contributors to libido loss, like stress and anxiety. Vitamins and minerals such as vitamin D, B vitamins, iron, and zinc play significant roles in mood regulation and mental clarity. A deficiency in these nutrients might trigger mood swings and depressive symptoms, impeding sexual desire.

It's also worth mentioning the social and psychological aspects involved in dietary choices. Shared meals and cooking experiences can enhance emotional bonds between partners, further rejuvenating their intimate lives. Cooking together can promote communication, foster teamwork, and create a shared sense of accomplishment, reinforcing emotional intimacy.

As we move forward, it's essential to consider not just what we eat but also how we approach food. Being mindful of dietary habits can lead to more conscious decisions that impact both health and relationships. It's a step towards taking personal responsibility for one's wellbeing, enhancing not just physical health but emotional and relational dynamics as well.

Unpacking nutrition's role in sexual health highlights the importance of adopting balanced dietary practices. By prioritizing a nutrient-rich diet, individuals can lay the groundwork for improvement in both sexual desire and overall quality of life. In the broader scope of addressing lifestyle factors, nutrition remains a cornerstone, a critical sphere where changes can lead to profound benefits. Ultimately, understanding and implementing these nutritional insights equips readers with a holistic toolset, enabling them to better contend with libido loss and its intertwined challenges.

The journey doesn't end with recognising these correlations. As each individual's nutritional needs differ, it may be beneficial to consult with healthcare professionals or nutritionists. They can offer personalized advice, helping tailor dietary approaches to suit specific health goals. By doing so, one can more effectively support sexual health and pave the way towards revitalised intimacy.

## The Role of Sleep

Understanding the integral role of sleep in our daily lives goes well beyond a mere preference for rest and relaxation. Sleep is an essential pillar supporting not only our overall health but also our libido and relationship dynamics. When men face a decline in sexual desire, it's often attributed to several lifestyle factors, one of which is increasingly recognised as an inadequate quality or quantity of sleep. In our journey to understand and address libido loss, we must highlight the multifaceted influence of sleep.

A restful night's sleep provides the body with an opportunity to replenish and rejuvenate, ensuring a balance of essential hormones such as testosterone, which plays a vital role in male libido. Testosterone levels inherently fluctuate throughout the day, typically peaking during the morning. However, insufficient or poor-quality sleep can disrupt this cycle, resulting in lower testosterone levels and consequently, a reduced sexual desire. Scientific studies have underscored this relationship, suggesting that men with restricted sleep patterns experience a significant decline in testosterone production.

Moreover, sleep deprivation doesn't just impact hormonal balance. It can also diminish cognitive function, leading to irritability, stress, and a dampening of mood—all of which can negatively influence intimate relationships. When you're tired, small irritations can become oversized issues. The resulting tensions can create a counterproductive cycle where unresolved conflicts further interrupt sleep, thereby exacerbating libido problems.

On top of this, chronic sleep issues such as insomnia or sleep apnoea can play a more insidious role. These conditions often lead to extended periods of reduced quality sleep, further compounding the strain on both physical health and emotional well-being. Addressing such issues should be a priority in restoring libido, as continuous sleep disruption has been linked to increased levels of stress hormones like cortisol, which can undermine sexual performance and intimacy.

Sleep also facilitates emotional regulation and mental clarity, elements that are crucial for maintaining the communication and empathy essential for healthy relationships. A good night's sleep equips individuals with the mental resilience to engage in effective dialogue, enabling couples to address issues collaboratively. When partners are rested, they're more likely to express empathy, show patience, and work together towards solutions for libido-related challenges.

So how can men and their partners harness sleep to revitalise their sexual health and relationships? Establishing a consistent sleep schedule is a good starting point. Try to go to bed and wake up at the same time each day, even on weekends, to support your body's natural circadian rhythms. This consistency reinforces your sleep-wake cycle, aiding in better quality rest and hormone regulation.

Creating a conducive sleep environment can also play a significant role. This includes investing in a comfortable mattress and pillows, maintaining a cool, dark bedroom, and eliminating noise disruptions. Limit exposure to screens and blue light close to bedtime, as these can interfere with the production of melatonin, the sleep hormone that signals your body to wind down.

Additionally, addressing lifestyle habits can make a profound difference. Regular physical activity, as discussed in other sections, enhances both sleep quality and sexual health, establishing a positive feedback loop. However, be mindful not to exercise too close to bedtime, as it might be too stimulating and interfere with your ability to fall asleep.

Consider relaxation techniques such as mindfulness or progressive muscle relaxation as part of your bedtime routine. These practices can help reduce anxiety and stress, promoting a peaceful transition into sleep. Incorporating such techniques can be particularly beneficial when dealing with underlying psychological contributors to libido decline, such as stress and anxiety, which are discussed in earlier chapters.

Furthermore, nutrition cannot be overlooked. Avoid caffeine and heavy meals close to bedtime, as these can disrupt sleep patterns. Alcohol, despite its initial sedative effects, can fragment sleep architecture and should be consumed with caution.

By prioritising sleep and understanding its profound connection to physical and emotional health, men can take a vital step in addressing declining libido. When approached as part of a comprehensive strategy that includes healthy lifestyle choices, open communication, and proactive problem-solving, sleep can become a powerful ally in restoring intimacy and passion.

In conclusion, the path to reigniting sexual desire and enhancing intimate relationships can seem daunting, with sleep just one piece of the puzzle. However, by acknowledging and addressing its role, we empower ourselves to reclaim both vitality and emotional connection. As with any lifestyle change, patience and persistence are key, but the rewards, as many have found, are well worth the effort.

## Substance Use and Misuse

Amidst the complexities of modern living, it's not uncommon for individuals to lean on substances—whether it be alcohol, tobacco, or recreational drugs—as a way to unwind or cope with life's challenges. However, the relationship between substance use and sexual desire can be a precarious one, often leading to unintended consequences. It's imperative to understand how these factors interplay with male libido, especially if there's a noticeable decline in your sexual drive.

The seduction of alcohol lies in its initial relaxing effects. A glass or two might seem to smooth social interactions and lower inhibitions, making it easier to engage with your partner. But there's a flipside, one that is scientifically backed. Excessive alcohol consumption can bring about a host of problems, including issues with sexual performance and libido. Chronic overindulgence may lead to hormonal imbalances, impacting testosterone levels which are crucial for maintaining a healthy sex drive. Binge drinking compounds these issues, leading not only to physiological consequences but potentially introducing emotional barriers between partners.

Equally concerning is the widespread use of tobacco products. Smoking is not only detrimental to one's health overall, but it specifically compromises cardiovascular function. Good blood flow is essential for sexual health, and when it's impaired, erectile difficulties may follow. These physical challenges are often accompanied by feelings of guilt or anxiety, which do no favours for sexual desire or intimacy. For those who are looking to enhance their sexual health, reducing or eliminating smoking from your lifestyle is a critical step.

Recreational drugs, while perceived by some as a means to enhance pleasure or escape, bring their own set of challenges. Substances like marijuana, ecstasy, or cocaine are known to initially heighten sensations, but with repeated use, they can dampen sexual desire and wreak havoc on relationship dynamics. Consistent usage often reshapes brain chemistry in ways that hinder normal sexual function, creating more obstacles in the pursuit of rekindling passion.

One of the often overlooked aspects of substance misuse is its psychological impact. Addiction—or even habitual use—can create dependency, prioritising the high over meaningful connections with partners. This shifting focus can lead to emotional strain in relationships, intensifying feelings of disconnect and reducing shared moments of intimacy. Partners may feel neglected or secondary to the substance, sparking conflict that further erodes sexual desire.

It's not just about curbing misuse but recognising when casual use tips into dependency territory. Self-awareness and honesty are crucial. Sometimes, the social pressure to indulge can run high, but understanding the trade-offs and taking a proactive stance toward moderation can significantly mitigate adverse effects on sexual health. Open dialogue with your partner about mutual concerns can be the foundation for a healthier, more conscious approach to substance use. Remember, it's less about eliminating all sources of enjoyment and more about finding a sustainable balance that supports both pleasure and wellbeing.

When looking to address substance use as a factor impacting libido, it's beneficial to explore lifestyle changes that reinforce positive habits. This might include integrating stress management techniques, like meditation or exercise, which serve not only to improve overall health but also to naturally boost libido. Focusing on a nutrient-rich diet, which fuels both mind and body, can play a role in reducing cravings and improving vitality.

And then there's the role of professional support. Encountering difficulty in addressing substance use on your own is far from unusual. Seeking help from therapists or addiction specialists can provide valuable tools and strategies. Such experts can guide you through understanding the root causes of substance dependence and develop coping mechanisms to overcome it. Often, therapy opens pathways to confront underlying psychological or emotional triggers that may be contributing to substance reliance.

Ultimately, making informed choices about substance use is a personal journey with profound implications for restoring and sustaining sexual desire. As you reflect on the place substances hold in your life, it may be helpful to consider how you wish to engage more fully with your partner, free from the barriers these substances may create. This is not just an individual quest, but one that can draw you and your partner closer, building support systems and intimacy without relying on external substances.

By focusing on moderation and exploring healthier alternatives, you can forge a path back to vibrant sexual health and a fulfilling relationship. Embracing this journey toward balance and mindfulness is a step toward reclaiming both your libido and the deeper connection with your partner that may seem elusive when under the shadow of substance misuse.

# Chapter 8:
# Reigniting Passion in Long-Term Relationships

Reigniting passion in long-term relationships requires more than a dash of romance; it demands a thoughtful rekindling of intimacy, understanding, and creativity. Couples can breathe new life into their connection by revitalising old customs and cultivating new rituals that foster closeness. This might be as simple as dedicating time for uninterrupted conversations, where partners rediscover each other's dreams or as exhilarating as exploring shared adventures that push boundaries and create lasting memories. Trust acts as the backbone of these efforts, reinforcing emotional security and openness. As couples venture into this journey of reignition, they'll find that with each step taken together, their partnership grows stronger and more resilient. Embracing vulnerability and maintaining a curious spirit allows for the creation of dynamic, enriching experiences that continuously kindle the flames of affection and attraction.

## Revitalising Romance

In long-term relationships, it's common for the initial spark to wane as the years go by. Life gets busy, routines become ingrained, and before you know it, the romance that once felt natural now requires a conscious effort to maintain. But don't despair; revitalising romance is within reach, and it's a journey that can be as fulfilling as the early days of love. The key is to infuse novelty into your relationship, explore shared passions, and communicate openly about your desires and expectations.

First and foremost, creating an atmosphere that flowers romance involves deliberate acts that might seem small but have profound effects. Consider how music can set the tone for an evening. Construct a playlist of songs that have meaning for both of you, or explore new music together. Lighting, too, can drastically change an environment. Soft, warm lights can make your home feel inviting and cosy, while scented candles can add a layer of sensory experience that heightens intimacy. This isn't about extravagant gestures; it's about making the effort to show your partner that they're cherished.

This process of rekindling love also invites openness to trying new things together. Think about activities that neither of you has tried before. It might be a dance class, a cooking workshop, or a weekend hiking trip. The act of engaging in these new experiences together can build a shared history, strengthen your bond, and offer fresh perspectives on each other. Importantly, these activities encourage you to step out of your comfort zones, creating a sense of adventure reminiscent of when your relationship was new.

Communication remains paramount. When talking to your partner about revitalising your romantic life, be open and honest about your needs. Share your thoughts without fear of judgment or dismissal, and encourage your partner to do the same. This dialogue is a delicate dance, involving both speaking and listening. By fostering an environment of emotional safety, you can express desires that may have felt hidden before, which can lead to deeper intimacy and understanding.

Surprise can be a powerful tool in bringing magic back to a relationship. Small surprises, like a handwritten note, a spontaneous outing, or a favourite meal prepared without occasion, can speak volumes about your affection. These acts don't just brighten the day;

they show that you're thinking of each other, and this ongoing investment in your relationship pays dividends in closeness and warmth.

Furthermore, intimacy isn't confined to grand gestures. It's also found in the quiet, everyday interactions—a gentle touch, a glance across a crowded room, a shared inside joke. These small moments of connection form the fabric of what binds you together, particularly as the initial passion evolves into a deeper, more sustainable love. Reflect on these moments and cherish them, for they're the heartbeat of romance.

Of course, physical closeness plays a crucial role in maintaining emotional connection. Explore different ways to be physically intimate beyond the sexual act itself—holding hands on a walk, cuddling on the sofa, or giving each other a massage. These actions can alleviate stress, promote trust, and renew the sense of togetherness that sometimes gets lost in everyday life.

Rekindling romance is not a one-time fix but an ongoing commitment to nurturing your relationship. Set aside regular time for each other, whether it's a weekly date night or a simple ritual that you both enjoy. This regularity can serve as a reminder of the love you share and a promise to continue growing together. Romance, in its most authentic form, is about appreciation and gratitude, being present in the moment, and celebrating the love that you've built together.

Nurturing romance in a long-term relationship is both an art and a science. It requires understanding your partner deeply and showing that you care in ways that resonate with them specifically. Reflect on what originally drew you to one another and find ways to appreciate these traits anew. Accept that relationships evolve and that each phase offers its own unique opportunities for connection and pleasure. With patience, creativity, and a genuine desire to connect, revitalising romance can transform your partnership, infusing it with new life and energy.

## Building Trust and Intimacy

Reigniting passion in long-term relationships isn't just about stoking the flames of romance; it's about nurturing a deep-rooted trust and intimacy that paves the way for genuine connection. Trust serves as the bedrock upon which every satisfying and enduring relationship is built, while intimacy adds layers of richness and nuance. When trust is compromised, intimacy can become elusive, and passion might wane. Thus, focusing on these integral aspects can enable couples to rekindle the fervour that initially brought them together.

Trust begins with transparency. Opening up about one's vulnerabilities, fears, and aspirations can be daunting, yet it's essential for building trust. Authentic communication fosters a sense of security and reliability—qualities that are paramount in long-term relationships. Intimacy thrives in an environment where both partners feel safe to express themselves genuinely without fear of judgement or betrayal.

It's vital to develop communication habits that enhance trust. Simple changes, like actively listening and validating your partner's experiences, can make a world of difference. When partners feel heard, they're more inclined to reciprocate, thus establishing a cycle of trust and mutual understanding. Active listening involves paying attention to what your partner says, responding empathically, and sometimes reading between the lines. This kind of engagement demonstrates that you value their thoughts and feelings and that you're invested in their well-being.

Intimacy isn't solely about physical closeness; it's also about connecting on an emotional and mental level. Shared experiences and activities can strengthen emotional bonds, allowing couples to rediscover each other's unique qualities. Engaging in new hobbies or traveling to unexplored places can invigorate the relationship, providing fresh perspectives and unique memories that can reignite the passion that's ebbed over time.

The physical aspect of intimacy, while important, is intertwined with emotional closeness. Building trust involves fostering an unconditional acceptance of your partner, which often translates into a more fulfilling physical connection. When both partners are secure in the relationship, they can more freely explore their desires and boundaries, leading to a more satisfying and balanced intimate life.

Of course, misunderstandings and disagreements are inevitable in any long-term partnership. However, how these are managed can significantly affect trust and intimacy. Constructive conflict resolution, rather than avoidance or escalation, is key. Approaching disputes with the intent to understand and resolve rather than to win can bring about positive outcomes. This mindset helps to reinforce the safety of the relationship, showing both partners that even during disagreement, their relationship remains strong and valued.

Moreover, recognising and appreciating each other's contributions within the relationship affirms the bond you share. Simple acknowledgements and expressions of gratitude can illuminate the path back to trusting intimacy. When both partners feel appreciated, they're likely to invest more in the relationship, knowing their efforts are valued. This reciprocation strengthens the trust and intimacy between them, bolstering their connection.

Trust and intimacy are dynamic and evolving. As couples progress through different stages of their relationship, these elements must be continuously nurtured and refined. Building a firm foundation early on isn't enough; consistent effort to maintain and grow these aspects is essential. This might involve setting aside regular time to discuss not just the logistics of life, but also personal dreams, concerns, and aspirations. These discussions can deepen understanding and bring couples closer.

Finally, it's crucial to remember that trust, once breached, can be rebuilt with effort and commitment. It might take time, and it's not always linear, but the rewards of persevering far outweigh the challenges. Intimacy can bloom anew when both partners are willing to open up, forgive past grievances, and focus on rebuilding their connection piece by piece.

## Creating New Experiences

In long-term relationships, one of the most thrilling pursuits is the creation of new experiences. It's not merely about altering routines or trying something different, but about reconnecting with your partner in ways that refresh your mutual intimacy. New experiences serve as a powerful catalyst, breathing life into what may have become predictable patterns of interaction. When couples engage in new activities together, they foster an environment ripe for growth, learning, and rediscovery. This process can effectively reignite passion by reminding each partner of the intrigue and curiosity that first sparked their interest in one another.

Exploring new experiences starts with a willingness to step outside the comfort zone, which can initially seem daunting. Yet, it's often in these uncharted territories that couples find the excitement and novelty that reignite their bond. Consider the array of possibilities— whether it's travelling to an undiscovered locale, taking up a new hobby together, or even engaging in spontaneous and playful activities. What's important is the shared intention to revive connection through fresh and invigorating encounters. While the activities themselves are significant, it's the shared commitment and effort that truly fuel the rekindling of romance.

Creating new experiences isn't limited to grand gestures or extravagant plans. Simple adjustments in routine or environment can be profoundly impactful. Perhaps it's as straightforward as a leisurely evening walk at an unusual time or a picnic in the living room with homemade treats and a classic film. Such activities, seemingly minor, can inspire candid conversations and laughter, both integral to sustaining a vibrant relationship. The act of breaking away from the ordinary routine can help couples see each other in a new light, rediscovering quirks and qualities that made them fall in love.

Sometimes, discovering new experiences involves learning more about oneself and one's partner—beyond what is already known. It might mean enrolling in a dance class or a cooking course, where both partners are students in the same journey of discovery. Here, success isn't measured in expertise but in shared experience and understanding. It's about recognising cues and signals from your partner, celebrating achievements together, and finding joy in each other's company. This partnership in learning encourages intimacy and reinforces the emotional connection that is foundational in long-term relationships.

Moreover, while new experiences can enhance physical connection, they equally touch on emotional and intellectual intimacy. Deep conversations spurred by indulging in something new can nurture mutual respect and admiration, creating a deeper and more resilient bond. Often, these dialogues uncover perspectives and insights about one another that may not surface in routine interactions. A relationship dynamic built on an understanding of emotional complexity is more likely to weather the inevitable challenges that come with time.

For many couples, shared adventures also offer the chance to test trust and reliance on each other. This trust-building exercise is pivotal as it encourages partners to support each other, showing vulnerability in trying circumstances or unknown activities. This vulnerability, far from being a weakness, actually strengthens the relationship, demonstrating the confidence and faith each partner has in the other. It's this secure foundation that allows couples to truly enjoy the new experiences they pursue, unencumbered by fears of judgement or failure.

In some cases, injecting novelty into a relationship can involve an element of playfulness and spontaneity. Reclaiming the youthful exuberance present at the beginning of a relationship can be a powerful way to reintroduce excitement. Playful activities—whether they involve friendly competition, such as playing a board game, or collaborative experiences like building something together—serve as a reminder of mutual fondness and enjoyment beyond adult responsibilities and stressors. This playfulness rekindles the thrill of early romance, a critical aspect of maintaining the spark over the years.

Conversely, new experiences do not always need to be joint endeavors. Encouraging and exploring individual passions and pursuits can bring back excitement and fresh perspectives into the relationship. When partners engage in activities they are passionate about, they are happier and more fulfilled, which naturally reflects in the relationship. Supporting each other's independent experiences can also underline the trust and respect in the partnership, key ingredients in any loving relationship.

As with any attempts at revitalisation, overcoming resistance is a common hurdle. Inertia and habitual comfort can often keep couples from endeavouring these new experiences. It's essential to communicate openly about any apprehensions or resistance, choosing activities that respect both partners' comfort levels and interests. The intention shouldn't be to push boundaries unreasonably, but to enrich the shared narrative with carefully chosen additions that align with mutual desires and aspirations.

Finally, it's crucial to take the time to enjoy and reflect on these experiences. Discussing what worked, what was enjoyed, and how it enhanced the connection can be as rewarding as the activities themselves. These reflections help consolidate the emotional benefits derived from new experiences, reinforcing positive memories and catalysing further connections. This ongoing process of creation and reflection is key to sustaining long-term intimacy and excitement.

In conclusion, the quest to create new experiences in a long-term relationship is a rewarding endeavour that requires both partners to embrace change and exploration. It's an essential component in the toolkit for reigniting passion, offering boundless opportunities to experience shared joy and tenderness. Whether through grand adventures or small, intimate changes, it's the pursuit of togetherness in varied forms that transforms relationships, reminding each partner of the infinite possibilities that arise from their connection. By weaving new experiences into the fabric of daily life, couples can continually reaffirm their love and commitment, keeping their relationship vibrant and resilient through the years.

# Chapter 9:
# Understanding the Female Perspective

In our journey to rekindle passion and navigate through the complexities of dwindling libido, it's pivotal to embrace the female perspective within relationships. Women often view emotional intimacy and sexual connection as intertwined, making understanding their perspective vital for reigniting passion. Establishing effective communication with your partner can bridge gaps and encourage a safe space for dialogue, fostering empathy and mutual understanding. Recognising the importance of listening and valuing each other's experiences can lead to collaborative problem-solving, ensuring both parties feel heard and respected. By nurturing a partnership built on open communication, empathy, and mutual goals, you're laying the groundwork for stronger connections and a reinvigorated intimate life that honours both partners' needs and desires.

## Effective Communication with Partners

Understanding the female perspective often begins with honing the skill of effective communication. It's not just about talking, but truly listening and engaging in a dialogue that values both parties' perspectives. Now, when it comes to the issue of libido decline and its impact on intimacy, conversations can sometimes feel daunting. The challenge is establishing a connection that invites openness and honesty without fear of judgement or rejection.

Men experiencing a dip in sexual desire might shy away from discussions that involve vulnerability. However, this hesitance can lead to misunderstandings and increased emotional distance. It's crucial to establish a communication style that encourages both partners to express their thoughts and feelings freely. Effective communication isn't simply about the exchange of words; it's the sincere effort to understand your partner's needs and empathetically share your own.

Starting such conversations when emotions are high may not be the best strategy. Instead, choose a moment of calm when both of you can engage without distractions or heightened emotions. Sometimes, this means setting aside a specific time where you can focus solely on each other. An intentional approach to dialogue not only shows commitment but also breeds a sense of safety and respect.

In the midst of these conversations, remember that your partner's emotions are valid. Often, libido issues may come with a sense of inadequacy or fear of change from both sides. It helps to reassure your partner that this is a journey you're not undertaking alone. The mutual understanding of this emotional landscape is pivotal. Active listening, a keystone of effective communication, will allow your partner to feel acknowledged and understood.

How do you listen actively? Start by giving your partner your full attention. This means putting away your phone, turning off the television, and maintaining eye contact. Show that you're engaged by nodding or giving verbal affirmations. Importantly, resist jumping in with solutions or defences. Instead, first seek to fully appreciate what your partner is expressing. This kind of attentive listening can transform a standard conversation into an opportunity for deeper connection and empathy.

Moreover, ask open-ended questions that encourage elaboration. Rather than questions that warrant a simple yes or no, engage with inquiries like, "How do you feel about this?" or "What do you think could help us move forward?" Such questions open doors to intricate and meaningful discussions, creating space for both partners to dive deeper into their feelings and thoughts.

It's natural to have conflicting perspectives. Yet, it's important to approach these differences with a spirit of curiosity rather than confrontation. Communicate with the intention of understanding rather than proving a point. This shift from adversarial to collaborative communication can guide the conversation towards common ground and shared goals.

Use "I" statements to express personal feelings and thoughts without placing blame. For instance, saying "I feel worried when..." as opposed to "You make me uncomfortable by..." reorients the dialogue towards your own experiences. This approach can help avoid defensive reactions while clearly stating your needs or concerns.

Avoid pitfalls like interrupting or raising your voice. These actions can escalate tension and deter honest communication. Instead, show respect and patience. Recognise that effective communication is often about quality, not quantity. Sometimes, a few minutes of genuine dialogue can be more impactful than hours of disconnected chatter.

Furthermore, it's crucial to address non-verbal cues in communication. Body language, tone of voice, and facial expressions all convey messages that words might not. Pay attention to your partner's non-verbal signals and be mindful of your own. Sometimes, a gentle touch or a reassuring smile can go a long way in bridging emotional gaps.

Sustainable communication also involves a degree of compromise. It's about finding a balance that honours both partners' needs. When discussing ways to tackle libido loss, be ready to explore solutions collaboratively, recognising that flexibility and sensitivity to each other's boundaries and preferences are key.

Remember to periodically assess your communication methods. Relationships are dynamic, and what worked yesterday might need adjustment today. Regularly touching base with your partner about how you both communicate can uncover areas needing growth and highlight what's working well, reinforcing the teamwork aspect of your partnership.

Ultimately, effective communication with partners is less about mastering a set technique and more about nurturing a mindset of openness and compassion. When both partners feel heard and valued, the intimacy lost to misunderstandings or misconceptions can begin to rebuild. Together, by cultivating this foundation, couples can navigate the challenges associated with libido decline and reinforce the bonds of their relationship, paving the way for renewed passion and connection.

## Empathy and Mutual Understanding

Empathy and mutual understanding lie at the heart of truly comprehending the female perspective, especially when addressing issues like libido loss. Building empathy involves stepping into your partner's shoes and comprehending their experiences without judgement. It's about recognising her emotions, thoughts, and feelings, and acknowledging them as valid. When you embark on this journey hand in hand, it can lead to transformative changes in your relationship. It's not only about resolving issues but also about deepening your connection and understanding.

The dynamics between partners when libido concerns arise can often become tangled in misunderstanding or assumptions. One partner might feel inadequate or undesired, while the other is struggling with internal conflicts that have nothing to do with their love or attraction. When empathy serves as your guide, it becomes possible to navigate these murky waters with clarity and patience. Understanding her perspective doesn't mean you need to be an expert on what she feels but rather an attentive and caring listener. Sometimes, simply being present and showing you care about her experience is enough to foster mutual understanding.

Effective communication is pivotal in nurturing empathy. It's imperative to create a safe, open environment where both partners feel comfortable expressing their needs and concerns. Start by asking open-ended questions and genuinely listening to her answers. Don't interrupt or rush to offer solutions, as sometimes what she needs most is not a fix, but a sympathetic ear. These dialogues can highlight areas of misunderstanding and allow both partners to explore what each other truly feels, promoting a shared comprehension.

Mutual understanding blossoms through shared experiences. Engage in activities that allow you both to reconnect and remind yourselves of what initially brought you together. Whether it's taking a stroll during sunset, cooking a meal together, or simply enjoying a quiet evening at home, these moments foster closeness and invite empathy naturally. As you cherish these moments together, you'll gain new insights into each other's worlds and see things from her viewpoint more clearly.

One of the key ingredients in cultivating empathy is patience. Intimacy and libido concerns might not resolve overnight, and that's perfectly okay. When you're patient, it affirms your commitment to the relationship and to her well-being. It's about acknowledging that the path you're on isn't linear, and embracing the ups and downs as part of your shared journey. You're in this together, and fostering mutual understanding means recognising that setbacks are merely stepping stones in the grander scheme of growth.

Recognising the unique differences in how men and women might perceive emotional and physical intimacy is crucial. Society often conditions women to prioritise emotional connection as a precursor to physical intimacy. Understanding this can illuminate why she might seem distant or disconnected if emotional needs aren't being met. In turn, this insight allows you to address underlying issues with empathy rather than frustration. It's not merely a problem to be solved but an opportunity to recalibrate your shared intimacy and grow stronger together.

Moreover, empathy flourishes through vulnerability. When both partners share their insecurities, fears, and desires without fear of judgment, it opens a window to true understanding. Mutual vulnerability cultivates a safe space where both of you know you can speak openly and truthfully, strengthening the foundation of your relationship. By laying your cards on the table, you both demonstrate a willingness to understand and be understood—a cornerstone of any lasting partnership.

Consider the role that cultural narratives and stereotypes play in shaping perceptions of libido and intimacy. Unpacking these can help both of you understand any preconceived notions that might influence your relationship. By challenging these stereotypes together, you pave the way for a more nuanced and satisfying intimate life. When empathy and mutual understanding drive this conversation, you're more likely to create an environment where both partners feel seen, heard, and valued.

Another aspect to consider is recognising and respecting boundaries. As you strive for mutual understanding, it's essential not to overstep in your eagerness to help or solve problems. Allow her the space to articulate her boundaries and be ready to respect them wholly. This respect is a profound form of empathy—it shows her that you value her autonomy and feelings. She'll be more likely to open up when she knows that her boundaries will be honoured.

Finally, remind yourselves that empathy and mutual understanding are ongoing practices rather than destinations. As you continue to nurture these attributes within your relationship, the rewards will ripple outward, enriching your intimate life and strengthening your emotional connection. Empathy encourages kindness and compassion, and when mutual understanding becomes the norm, it fosters resilience in the face of life's inevitable challenges. Together, you can navigate the complexities of libido loss not just with love, but with a deep-seated respect for each other's unique experiences and perspectives.

## Collaborative Problem Solving

Understanding a partner's perspective isn't just an inherent ability; it's a skill that, when honed, can transform relationships, especially when navigating the complexities of libido loss. Engaging in collaborative problem solving offers couples an opportunity to jointly address the challenges that arise when sexual desire wanes. This approach encourages mutual respect, shared goals, and open communication, all critical factors in revitalising a relationship.

In most relationships, the issue of diminished libido doesn't occur in isolation. It's wrapped in layers of emotional complexity, making it essential to approach solutions collectively. Acknowledging that both partners may experience frustration, confusion, or even guilt can diffuse tension and pave the way for a more cooperative atmosphere. Partners who can empathise with each other's feelings are better equipped to devise workable solutions that respect each partner's boundaries, needs, and desires.

An effective starting point for collaborative problem solving is creating an environment where both partners feel comfortable expressing their innermost thoughts. Such a space fosters honesty and vulnerability, essential for understanding the unique challenges and emotional landscapes each partner navigates. Communication is key, but it's effective communication that lays the groundwork for successful collaboration. Partners should practice active listening, a technique that involves fully concentrating, understanding, and responding thoughtfully to each other.

Empathy plays a vital role in this process. When a partner genuinely seeks to understand what their counterpart is going through, it diminishes feelings of isolation. Sharing perspectives and being open to compromise are integral steps in building a collaborative framework. It's important to recognise that differing perceptions may exist, and these differences needn't be points of contention but instead topics for exploration and growth.

Collaborative problem solving in relationships doesn't mean merging into one entity; rather, it involves maintaining individual identities while working towards common goals. The individuality each partner brings to the equation can enrich problem-solving efforts. By pooling diverse perspectives, couples can create innovative solutions they might not have arrived at domestically. Moreover, this teamwork can strengthen their emotional connection, furthering the sense of unity.

A practical approach to fostering collaboration involves identifying shared objectives and aspirations for the relationship. To reinvigorate desire, it can be helpful for partners to discuss what intimacy means to them and what shifts they hope to see. This dialogue sets a foundation upon which joint action plans can be built. Incorporating structured tools, such as goal-setting and progress tracking, can make dreams of rekindled passion more tangible and achievable.

Aside from emotional and communicative strategies, taking collaborative action often involves a willingness to adapt behaviours and routines. This might mean scheduling regular date nights or actively participating in each other's hobbies to build emotional closeness. It's also beneficial to explore activities that neither partner has tried before, encouraging a sense of adventure and novelty. Such experiences can reignite a sense of partnership and shared achievement.

Nevertheless, it's crucial for couples to monitor and evaluate the impact of their collaborative efforts periodically. Open and honest feedback sessions provide a forum where both partners can express satisfaction or concerns regarding their progress. These sessions aren't about assigning blame but rather about adjusting strategies to better align with their evolving needs.

Recognising when external support might be beneficial is another key aspect of collaborative problem solving. While many couples can navigate through the troughs of libido loss independently, others may feel the need to consult therapists or counsellors who specialise in intimacy and sexual health. Reaching out for guidance doesn't signal failure but demonstrates a commitment to cultivating a healthier and happier relationship.

In summary, embracing collaborative problem solving requires an understanding that solutions rarely come packaged in singular formulas. It's an ongoing, dynamic process that demands both commitment and creativity from both partners. By forging a path together, partners not only address the immediate issue of declining libido but also fortify their relationship against future challenges. This collaborative journey, rich with empathy, communication, and mutual understanding, can transform how partners engage with each other and renew the passionate connection they've longed to rekindle.

# Chapter 10:
## Navigating Medical Treatments

Navigating the landscape of medical treatments for libido loss can feel overwhelming, but it offers a promising path towards restoring intimacy. Understanding the role of commonly used medications is crucial; they can be effective when employed appropriately under medical supervision. Beyond conventional medicines, alternative therapies present viable options that range from herbal supplements to holistic approaches. It's essential, however, to approach these with discernment, as not all alternative treatments boast equivalent efficacy. This journey mandates proactive dialogue with healthcare professionals who can provide tailored advice, ensuring decisions align with personal health profiles and goals. By building a collaborative relationship with your medical provider, you not only access expert insights but also contribute to mapping out a well-informed strategy for addressing these challenges. The road to revitalised desire requires delving not merely into medication, but also into a broader understanding of available options, empowering individuals to make informed choices and embrace hope for renewing passion and connection.

## Commonly Used Medications

When it comes to addressing issues with libido, particularly for men experiencing a noticeable decline, medications can often be a viable option. They can provide relief and potentially reignite the spark in one's intimate life. While medications shouldn't be the first line of defence, they can be an essential part of a comprehensive approach to enhancing sexual desire, especially when lifestyle changes and psychological interventions need further support.

Phosphodiesterase type 5 inhibitors, or PDE5 inhibitors, have become household names in discussions surrounding men's sexual health. Viagra (sildenafil), Cialis (tadalafil), and Levitra (vardenafil) are some popular choices. Primarily prescribed to tackle erectile dysfunction, these medications help increase blood flow to the penis, facilitating easier attainment and maintenance of erections. Interestingly, their effectiveness has a side benefit of enhancing overall sexual confidence, which can indirectly help revitalize libido. However, it's crucial to remember these medications don't stimulate desire on their own—psychological and emotional readiness still play significant roles.

Testosterone replacement therapy (TRT) is another avenue worth exploring, especially for those with clinically low testosterone levels. Testosterone influences many biological functions, including libido, energy levels, and mood. Restoring testosterone to its normal range can lead to significant improvements in sexual interest and performance. However, this therapy requires careful medical supervision due to potential side effects, such as an increased risk of cardiovascular issues and prostate problems. Regular monitoring and a personalised approach are advisable when considering TRT.

The world of medication isn't limited to oral options. Topical treatments exist, delivering hormones like testosterone directly through the skin. These include gels and patches, which can provide a steady release of testosterone, aiding in libido restoration safely. The choice between oral or topical should be guided by factors like personal preference, medical history, and lifestyle considerations. Consulting with a healthcare provider is essential to determine the most suitable and effective option for individual needs.

*Find a balance,* some might say, is key when it comes to managing libido loss. While medications can offer significant benefits, reliance solely upon them without addressing underlying causes can lead to a cycle of dependency and disappointing results. Incorporating psychological support or counseling to complement medication use can ensure a holistic approach, addressing both the symptoms and root causes of libido decline.

Antidepressants and anxiety medications also deserve mention, but with caution. SSRIs (selective serotonin reuptake inhibitors) are commonly prescribed for depression and anxiety, but a well-known side effect is a potential decrease in sexual desire. Not all individuals experience this, but if you're considering or are already on these medications, it's critical to discuss with your doctor the possibility of sexual side effects. Sometimes, adjusting the dosage or exploring alternative medications can alleviate unwanted impacts on your libido.

Surprisingly, some lesser-known medications have surfaced as off-label options for enhancing libido. For instance, bupropion, typically prescribed for depression, has shown potential in improving sexual desire without the adverse libido effects often associated with other antidepressants. As with any medical treatment, achieving the right outcome involves collaborative conversation with a healthcare professional to tailor choices specifically for you.

Ultimately, navigating medications in the pursuit of libido restoration involves weighing benefits against risks, understanding personal health priorities, and ensuring a personalised approach to treatment. It's about restoring not just physical function but enhancing life quality and intimate connections. The journey through medications, when complemented with lifestyle changes and relationship dynamics adjustments, can lead to profound, positive transformations in one's intimate life.

## Alternative Therapy Options

Navigating the world of medical treatments can sometimes feel overwhelming, especially when considering the multitude of options available for addressing a decline in sexual desire. However, alongside conventional medicines, alternative therapies have emerged as a viable path for those seeking a more holistic approach to reigniting passion and intimacy. These therapies focus on the interconnectedness of mind, body, and spirit, offering solutions that go beyond mere symptom management.

One of the most talked-about alternative therapies is acupuncture. Originating from ancient Chinese medicine, acupuncture involves inserting thin needles into specific points on the body. The aim is to balance the body's energy, or "qi", which can enhance overall well-being. It's suggested that acupuncture might help with libido loss by relieving stress and promoting relaxation, creating a more conducive mental state for intimacy. Some preliminary studies have shown promising results, linking acupuncture to improved sexual function and satisfaction. However, the effectiveness of this treatment can vary widely, and it is crucial to seek a licensed and experienced practitioner.

Herbal medicine also offers a range of solutions that appeal to those looking to avoid pharmaceuticals. Ginseng, for instance, has been traditionally used in many cultures as a natural libido booster. Studies have indicated that ginseng might influence the central nervous system and encourage hormonal balance, potentially boosting sexual desire. Another herb, Maca root, grown mainly in Peru, has been associated with increased fertility and libido. As with all herbal treatments, it's essential to approach them with caution and consult healthcare professionals, particularly regarding dosage and potential interactions with other medications.

Another intriguing option is the use of aromatherapy. This practice involves the use of essential oils, extracted from various plants, which are either inhaled or applied to the skin. Some essential oils, such as ylang-ylang, rose, and sandalwood, are reputed for their aphrodisiac properties. These scents can help create a relaxing, sensual atmosphere that may support increased sexual desire by reducing anxiety and promoting emotional connection between partners.

Homeopathy is another alternative approach that resonates with many. Based on the principle of treating "like with like", homeopathy employs highly diluted substances to trigger the body's self-healing response. While critics often question the scientific basis of homeopathy, some individuals attest to its effectiveness in revitalising libido. Remedies like Lycopodium and Natrum Muriaticum are often suggested, tailored to the individual's unique symptoms and emotional state.

Yoga and meditation are powerful tools that more and more people are turning to for managing stress and enhancing overall health. The practise of yoga combines postures, breathing exercises, and meditation. It strengthens the mind-body connection, which can improve body awareness and reduce stress levels. Certain yoga poses, such as the Cobra Pose and the Bridge Pose, are believed to stimulate the pelvic region, potentially enhancing sexual energy and desire. On the other hand, meditation encourages mindfulness and presence, qualities that enhance the art of intimacy by allowing individuals to be more attuned to their own needs and those of their partner.

One mustn't overlook the potential impact of dietary changes. While this might lean more towards a lifestyle factor, certain diets or nutritional practices are often considered alternative in nature. A focus on natural, whole foods, free from chemical additives, can create an environment in which the body feels invigorated and balanced. Meanwhile, incorporating foods rich in omega-3 fatty acids, such as salmon or flaxseed, can support cardiovascular health and, by extension, improve sexual performance.

Mind-body therapies such as Tai Chi and Qigong are gaining popularity as well. These practices combine movement, meditation, and breathing exercises to promote mental and physical health. They aim to enhance the vital energy within the body, which can help improve clarity of mind and emotional stability, contributing to a healthier sexual life.

Hypnotherapy is yet another intriguing option. It works on the subconscious mind, often helping individuals overcome psychological barriers linked to sexual dysfunction. By using guided relaxation and focused attention, hypnotherapy seeks to change pre-existing negative thought patterns and reinforce positive behaviours. For some, this intervention can be transformative, offering clarity and a renewed sense of confidence in their ability to connect deeply with their partner.

Biofeedback, though less mainstream, is a method that teaches control over certain physiological functions. Through biofeedback, individuals can learn to regulate aspects like muscle tension and heart rate. This management of stress responses can, in turn, lead to a relaxed state, which is crucial for a healthy sex drive.

It's important to remember that while alternative therapies offer diverse avenues for overcoming libido challenges, they are not a one-size-fits-all solution. What works wonders for one might not be effective for another, necessitating a personal experimentation phase. The journey entails exploring various methods, keeping an open mind, and maintaining insight into how different treatments align with one's values and lifestyle.

The choice to pursue alternative therapy for libido loss should be made carefully and in consultation with a healthcare provider. Ensuring that these methods complement any existing treatments is key to a safe and effective recovery journey. As you embark on this path, let curiosity and self-compassion guide you. Embrace the potential for growth and renewal these therapies can bring, while acknowledging the interconnectedness of the body and mind as you strive to rekindle passion and deepen the intimate connection with your partner.

## Seeking Medical Advice

For many men experiencing a decline in sexual desire, seeking medical advice can be a daunting yet essential step. It offers a pathway to understanding underlying causes and developing a tailored approach to remedy the situation. Many prefer to tackle issues privately or believe that a drop in libido is something they must endure alone. However, reaching out to a healthcare professional can unravel complexities that might be difficult to navigate independently. The act of seeking professional guidance not only aids in finding effective treatments but can also provide peace of mind.

Understanding what to expect from a consultation can help ease apprehensions. During an initial appointment, a thorough assessment of medical history is likely. This process often delves into lifestyle habits, mental health, and any medications being taken, all of which can influence sexual wellness. A doctor might inquire about specific symptoms, changes in libido, and emotional well-being. Being open and honest here can significantly enhance the quality of care received. Remember, confidentiality and professionalism are core responsibilities of healthcare providers. You're in a space where speaking candidly enables precise analysis and, consequently, more effective treatment options.

For the medical professional, the aim is often to rule out or identify medical conditions that could be affecting sexual desire. Conditions such as diabetes, heart disease, or endocrine disorders are known to intersect with libido levels. Blood tests might be performed to assess hormone levels, particularly testosterone, which plays a pivotal role in sexual desire. Depending on the findings, further tests might be suggested to gather more detailed insights. The key takeaway here is that addressing a medical root cause not only aids libido but can also improve overall health.

Discussing potential treatment avenues is a critical component of seeking medical advice. Depending on the diagnosis, medication might be recommended. There are several medications designed to address libido issues and sexual functionality. It is crucial to understand how each medication works, its side effects, and how it interacts with any current prescriptions. Armed with this knowledge, you and your doctor can weigh risks and benefits, ensuring the chosen treatment aligns with your lifestyle and goals.

Apart from conventional medical treatments, discussions might extend to include alternative therapies. These can encompass anything from herbal supplements to acupuncture. It's important to approach such options with a discerning mind and a sceptical eye, ensuring they complement rather than contradict conventional treatments. Your medical advisor can provide guidance on the safety and efficacy of such alternatives, helping to integrate them into a holistic treatment plan that considers both mind and body.

Consultations with specialists may be warranted in more complex cases. An endocrinologist, for instance, can offer deeper insights into hormonal dynamics, while a urologist might focus on structural or functional issues. Collaborating with specialists, your primary physician creates a comprehensive picture of your health, honing in on specific areas that require attention. Each specialist brings a unique perspective, contributing to a well-rounded treatment plan.

Beyond physical health, mental health professionals may also play a crucial role. Stress, anxiety, and depression are significant contributors to declining libido. Seeking help from a therapist or counsellor can provide strategies to manage these emotional burdens. Cognitive behavioural therapy, mindfulness practices, or stress-reduction techniques are some of the tools psychologists might employ to help recover sexual interest. Hospitals and clinics may offer holistic services, combining medical and psychological support under one roof.

Ultimately, the decision to seek medical advice should be viewed as a positive and empowering step. It signifies a commitment to reclaiming control over one's health and intimacy, potentially transforming personal and relational dynamics. Partners can be a supportive presence during medical consultations, ensuring that both parties understand the treatment path and share in the healing journey. Such shared experiences can strengthen the emotional bonds necessary for intimacy to thrive.

Fostering a collaborative approach with your healthcare provider is crucial. Ask questions, voice concerns, and engage with the options presented. An informed patient is a proactive patient, leading to more tailored and successful outcomes. As knowledge grows, so does the capacity to maintain and enhance libido in the face of life's varied challenges.

Remember, while medical advice is invaluable, it is part of a broader landscape that includes psychological, relational, and lifestyle considerations. Consistency and dedication to the process can yield substantial improvements over time. By persistently working alongside medical professionals, you'll not only strive for improved libido but also improve overall well-being and satisfy the journey to a more fulfilling intimate relationship.

# Chapter 11:
## The Power of Mindfulness

In the hustle of modern life, reconnecting with one's partner can be a challenge, often hindered by the mind darting between past regrets and future anxieties. Yet, mindfulness offers an empowering avenue to anchor oneself in the present, fostering deeper connections and enlivening dormant desire. By embracing the moment and letting go of distractions, men can tune into the subtleties of their emotional and physical landscapes, opening new pathways for intimacy. Mind-body connection techniques, such as mindful breathing and body scans, invite a harmonious awareness that breaks down barriers blocking passion. Regular meditative practices not only calm the restless mind but also pave the way for an enriched sense of togetherness and shared joy with one's partner. Through mindfulness exercises tailored for intimacy, couples can rediscover their unique rhythms, transforming daily interactions into meaningful and sensual experiences. This journey doesn't just reignite passion; it nurtures a more resilient bond, deepening emotional intimacy and laying a solid foundation for lasting fulfilment in their relationship.

## Mind-Body Connection Techniques

When you're facing a decline in sexual desire, it's easy to think of it as a purely physical challenge or blame it exclusively on stress or emotional disconnect. However, the interplay between the mind and body is the cornerstone of not just resolving libido issues but enhancing overall intimacy. Recognising and harnessing this connection can pave the way for meaningful change, inviting you and your partner to redefine your intimate experiences.

Mind-body connection techniques are centred on the premise that our thoughts, emotions, and physical states don't exist in isolation. Rather, they continuously influence each other, creating a dynamic where balance or imbalance in one aspect can affect the others. One way to tap into this connection is through *mindful breathing*, a practice that directs your focus to the rhythm of your breath, allowing you to ground yourself in the present moment. By doing so, you not only calm the mind but also create a ripple effect of relaxation and physiological harmony throughout the body.

Consider the role of **progressive muscle relaxation** as part of your mind-body toolkit. This technique involves systematically tensing and then slowly releasing different muscle groups. By doing so, you become more aware of the physical manifestations of tension and where they reside in your body. Through regular practice, you'll learn to release this tension more effectively, nurturing a state of calmness and receptiveness which is essential for sexual rediscovery.

Engaging in *visualisation* is another strategy that effectively bridges the gap between mind and body. By envisioning intimate scenarios that evoke positive emotions, both partners can vividly reconnect with sensations that might have become muted over time. This isn't about creating unrealistic fantasies but rather enhancing psychological arousal, making real-world sexual experiences more engaging and satisfying.

A significant part of healing and enhancing libido through the mind-body connection involves cultivating **self-awareness**. Journalling can be an incredibly powerful tool in this regard. By taking time each day to jot down thoughts and feelings, men can gain insights into their emotional triggers and the physical reactions that accompany them. This newfound understanding can then inform more conscious decisions around managing stress, enhancing mood, and fostering environments conducive to intimacy.

Let's shift our attention to the benefits of incorporating *yoga and tai chi* into your routine. These practices are celebrated not just for their physical benefits but for their ability to merge awareness, movement, and breath in a harmonious dance. Through regular practice, you're likely to see improvements in flexibility and endurance, but more crucially, they'll help you cultivate patience and presence—qualities that are inherently valuable in intimate relationships.

It's also worth exploring the influence of **biofeedback techniques** within this context. These train you to harness physiological activity for improved performance—the kind that isn't just beneficial in sports but equally transformative in addressing sexual challenges. By learning to control bodily responses such as heart rate and muscle tension, you build the groundwork for enhanced relaxation and control during sexual activity, fostering a deeply connected experience with your partner.

But beyond structured techniques, the mind-body connection thrives on simply being present. How often do we find ourselves distracted by screens or lost in thoughts of tomorrow? Practising *mindful presence*—whether during times of intimacy, shared activities, or even mundane moments—can significantly enhance your relationship. By giving full attention to your partner, you create an environment of respect and openness, facilitating an exchange of deeper emotional and physical connection.

In looking at practical steps, start small. Introduce five minutes of mindful breathing into your daily routine, gradual relaxation exercises before bed, or once-weekly yoga sessions. These might seem insignificant at first glance, but consistency in practice is where transformation gently unfolds. It's about instilling a habit of the mind-body connection rather than a hurried fix, fostering long-term changes in your sexual health and relationship dynamics.

Furthermore, don't underestimate the power of communication in strengthening these techniques. Share your experiences and progress with your partner, opening up discussions around both successes and areas of difficulty. Your journey of rediscovery can strengthen not just your personal connection but provide a shared narrative around growth and intimacy.

Above all, embrace compassion as you explore these techniques. It's easy to get caught up in performance or the need for quick results, but remember that this journey is personal and uniquely yours. The mind-body connection offers pathways to deeper understanding and rejuvenation; it's a reminder that you and your partner deserve an intimate life that's as emotionally satisfying as it is physically fulfilling.

As we continue to explore mindfulness, moving into meditative practices, and exercises specifically tailored for enhancing intimacy, you'll find an array of strategies to further invigorate your relationship. These techniques aren't just about addressing current struggles. They're about laying down the foundations for a more vibrant, connected, and fulfilling future.

## Meditative Practices

In a world teeming with distractions and responsibilities, the ability to centre one's mind and harness its potential can feel elusive. However, when it comes to restoring and nurturing sexual desire, the practices of meditation could hold the key. Meditative practices bring the promise of inner peace and reconnection, both within oneself and with one's partner. Practising meditation isn't merely about sitting cross-legged and chanting; it's an intentional journey into self-awareness and understanding, particularly when grappling with the complexities of libido loss.

Stepping into meditation is akin to stepping into a world where time slows, and the symphony of thoughts can finally be heard and managed. For men experiencing a decline in sexual desire, meditative practices provide a valuable tool for acknowledging and navigating the mental blocks that accompany this experience. It's about learning to listen to the body's needs and rhythms without judgement. As one embarks on this meditative path, the immediate goal is not to solve everything overnight but to gradually cultivate an environment where passion can thrive once more.

Engaging in meditation has been shown to reduce stress levels, a common contributor to libido decline. Stress isn't always external—often, it's the internal pressures we place upon ourselves that weigh the heaviest. Through mindfulness meditation, one can learn to identify these stress-inducing thoughts and attitudes, gently steering the mind towards calmness. Short, guided sessions focusing on deep breathing and body scans can foster relaxation and help turn down the volume on mental noise, paving the way for enhanced focus and presence in intimate settings.

Meditative practices also serve as a bridge to deeper emotional intelligence. Understanding one's emotions and how they correlate with desires and actions can significantly impact sexual relationships. Consider mindfulness practices designed in empathy enhancement, such as loving-kindness meditation (or "metta" meditation), which encourages the cultivation of compassion, both towards oneself and others. This practice aids individuals in moving past self-criticism and towards a more loving dialogue within their relationships, building a foundation of trust and understanding critical for rekindling passion.

Furthermore, meditation provides a space to explore one's intentions and desires, liberating one from societal prescriptions and opening up channels for genuine self-expression. This exploration isn't about adhering to preconceived notions of sexual vitality but about discovering and honouring what genuinely ignites one's passion. By delving into quiet reflection and introspection through meditative practices, individuals may uncover new dimensions of their sexuality previously obscured by the cacophony of daily obligations and stress.

Incorporating meditative practices into daily routines needn't be daunting or overwhelming. Mindfulness can be seamlessly woven into everyday life through simple activities like mindful walking or eating, where each step or bite becomes an opportunity for awareness. By starting small, with perhaps just a few minutes dedicated to stillness, individuals can gradually build up to more extended sessions that delve deeper into the realms of consciousness and desire.

These practices aren't solely for individual gain. They can be a shared journey, strengthening relational bonds and aligning partners on a path towards mutual understanding and satisfaction. Pairing up for meditation sessions encourages open communication and vulnerability, fostering an atmosphere where intimacy thrives. Partners embarking on this journey together may find that their shared experiences in mindful practices create a profound and supportive connection, necessary for navigating the complexities of libido loss with empathy and creativity.

As individuals immerse themselves in meditation, they may discover an emerging sense of fulfilment and balance that extends beyond sexual desire. Mindful presence empowers individuals to live fully in moments, savour each experience anew, and approach challenges with calm curiosity. These qualities, naturally spilling into the intimacy shared with a partner, offer a transformative viewpoint, where love-making becomes an enriching experience rather than a performance or obligation.

Taking time for meditative practices is an investment in oneself and one's relationship. It's a commitment to personal growth and the flourishing of shared love. As men and their partners explore the possibilities meditational routines provide, they may find themselves more attuned to not only their needs but also to each other's, carving a path towards restored intimacy and enduring connection. Engaging in these practices is an invitation to embark on a lifelong journey of mindfulness, with passion and love serving as trusted companions along the way.

## Mindfulness Exercises for Intimacy

In the ever-evolving journey of maintaining closeness with a partner, mindfulness offers a pathway to deepen emotional and physical connection. It provides a bridge, encouraging both partners to be fully present and engaged with one another, enhancing every moment shared. Through the deliberate practice of mindfulness, couples can transform their interactions, cultivating a profound sense of intimacy that transcends the ordinary encounters of daily life.

Mindfulness, at its core, is about paying attention to the present moment without judgement. When applied to intimacy, this means being wholly present with your partner, both physically and emotionally. It's a process of rediscovering each other through a fresh lens, unclouded by past conflicts or future anxieties. As we navigate the complexities of relationships, particularly in long-term commitments, these exercises act as anchors, grounding partners in the now.

One of the simplest yet most effective mindfulness exercises for intimacy involves eye contact. Though seemingly straightforward, maintaining eye contact longer than usual, without speaking, can create an intense bond. This practice requires vulnerability, but it's in this vulnerability that trust and closeness blossom. Setting aside just five minutes a day for this exercise can gradually enhance how comfortable you feel with one another, dismantling walls that might have been built over time.

Next, consider the power of mindful touch. Our skin is a sensitive canvas capable of conveying warmth, affection, and security. Engaging in mindful touch involves focusing on the sensations in your fingertips as they meet your partner's skin. Be attentive to the texture, temperature, and contours you encounter. Instead of rushing through a tactile moment, linger. Allow your hands to communicate what words might struggle to express; tenderness, love, and devoted attention. This simple act can deepen emotional bonds and heighten physical pleasure.

Another practice is to embark upon a shared meditation session. Start with guided meditations tailored for couples or explore silent meditations where each partner mirrors the other's breath. This shared stillness cultivates a space of mutual understanding and synchronicity. Often, in silence, partners learn more about each other than they do through conversation. Such exercises encourage empathy, patience, and a deeper emotional connection, aligning both hearts and minds.

Incorporating gratitude reflections bolsters mindfulness with an additional layer of appreciation. At the end of the day, pause and reflect on what you appreciate about your partner. These can be small, everyday gestures or significant acts of kindness. Verbalise this gratitude, sharing your reflections with each other. This ritual fosters an environment of positivity, reminding both partners of the reasons they cherish one another, which effectively rekindles affection and mutual respect.

Then there's mindful listening, an essential skill to nurture intimacy. Too often, amidst the cacophony of modern life, we listen to respond rather than to understand. Mindful listening involves giving your partner your undivided attention, fully absorbing what they express without interrupting. Nod, ask clarifying questions, or reflect back what you've heard. This practice not only improves communication but also creates a safe space for sharing deeper emotions and thoughts, fortifying the connection you share.

Engaging in daily mindfulness walks can also serve as a bonding thread. Walking side by side, perhaps in nature, allows couples to harmonise their paces. Focus on the rhythmic sound of footsteps, the rustling leaves, or the chirping of birds, letting these moments of simplicity draw you closer. Such walks can open pathways to spontaneous conversations, enabling moments of laughter and rediscovery.

And finally, explore a sensory immersion exercise. This involves preparing a meal together, eating it mindfully, and engaging all five senses. Savour the flavours, feel the textures, notice the colours, listen to the crunch, and smell the aromas. Share your sensations with each other, discussing textures and tastes to foster a greater appreciation of the shared experience. This sensory mindfulness invites a playful exploration of pleasure, intensifying the joys of everyday life.

Each of these exercises encourages couples to explore intimacy through mindfulness, fostering a refreshed appreciation of each other. By implementing these practices, relationships can escape the mundane routines and renew passion and connection. It's a gentle reminder that true intimacy isn't about grand gestures but about being there, truly and fully, in each moment together.

Ultimately, mindfulness transforms how we perceive and experience intimacy, offering fresh insights into ourselves and our partners. It reminds us that while life constantly pushes forward, we can choose to pause, appreciate, and connect. Through mindful practices, couples can turn everyday interactions into profound, meaningful expressions of love and closeness, reigniting the flames of intimacy and passion.

In embracing mindfulness exercises for intimacy, couples find that the experiences shared are fuller, richer, and more satisfying. The world might be bustling around them, but inside their shared mindfulness, they find peace, presence, and a profound connection. In this transformative journey, intimacy becomes not just a part of life but a celebration of each other's essence, embraced fully with understanding, empathy, and love.

# Chapter 12:
## Overcoming Common Barriers

In the quest to rekindle a vibrant and fulfilling intimate relationship, many men and their partners face a myriad of barriers, each posing unique challenges yet offering opportunities for growth. While these roadblocks such as the fear of failure, self-perception challenges, and deeply ingrained misconceptions might seem daunting, it's crucial to confront and navigate through them with resilience and understanding. Fear of failure, for instance, can often cripple one's confidence, yet it also serves as a pivotal moment where re-evaluating personal expectations can lead to empowerment and renewed vigour. Meanwhile, self-perception challenges demand a compassionate reassessment of how one views themselves, offering the perfect chance to cultivate a healthier and more accepting self-image. Misconceptions, often shaped by societal pressures and misinformation, require dismantling through open dialogue and education, allowing a clearer path forward. Approaching these barriers not as insurmountable obstacles but as stepping stones can transform not only a man's relationship with himself but also with his partner, leading to a deeper, more meaningful connection. Through perseverance, reflection, and collaboration, overcoming these common barriers becomes not only feasible but transformative, laying the foundation for a renewed intimacy and shared joy.

## Fear of Failure

When we talk about libido, it's not just a matter of biological impulses or mental states; it's deeply intertwined with the fear of failure. This fear, often unacknowledged and lurking in the background, can significantly impede one's ability to enjoy a fulfilling intimate life. Men, especially, are conditioned to equate sexual prowess with success, making the stakes feel even higher. The fear of not living up to a partner's expectations or cultural standards can be paralysing, creating a cycle where anxiety leads to performance issues, which in turn exacerbates the fear.

This fear isn't merely psychological noise; it has real physiological implications. Stress and anxiety triggered by the fear of failure can lead to the release of cortisol, a hormone that in high amounts can negatively affect sexual health. It's a cruel irony that the anxiety about failing can directly contribute to the very outcomes one is most anxious about. This vicious cycle makes understanding and addressing the fear of failure crucial to overcoming barriers in one's intimate life.

Furthermore, the fear of failure can stifle open communication between partners. It isn't easy to admit vulnerabilities, especially when there's a looming sense of inadequacy. However, fostering a space where both partners feel safe to express concerns and fears without judgment can significantly alleviate this pressure. Open dialogue disrupts the silence surrounding these fears, allowing couples to work collaboratively toward solutions. Mutual support and reassurance can transform a relationship from a potential opponent to an ally in confronting these anxieties.

Embracing vulnerability is key to overcoming the fear of failure. It requires one to redefine what success means in the context of intimate relationships. Instead of striving for unrealistic standards, focusing on genuine connection and shared experiences can help shift the perspective from performance-based sexuality to one grounded in mutual respect and affection. This shift fosters a deeper intimacy that transcends mere physical encounters.

Positive reinforcement plays a pivotal role as well. Celebrating small victories rather than dwelling on perceived failures can change the narrative. It's about recognising progress, no matter how incremental, and understanding that intimacy is a journey, not a destination. Like the process of learning any new skill, it involves setbacks and crossings, but each step forward is a testament to resilience and growth.

Integrating mindfulness practices can also help dismantle the fear of failure by encouraging presence and acceptance. Techniques such as deep breathing and grounding exercises can enhance one's ability to stay present in the moment, reducing anxiety about outcomes and fostering a greater sense of peace and confidence. Practising mindfulness together with a partner can amplify these benefits, synchronising both individuals' emotional and physical states.

Moreover, understanding that fear of failure isn't an isolated issue, but rather a shared human experience, can be profoundly liberating. Many individuals grapple with similar anxieties, and recognising this normalcy can lessen the isolation often felt. Therapy and support groups provide spaces to explore these issues collectively, offering insights and strategies from those who have navigated similar challenges.

Ultimately, dismantling the fear of failure requires patience, perseverance, and a willingness to redefine personal and relational goals. By confronting and understanding this fear, individuals and couples can carve pathways to profound intimacy and fulfilment, finding strength and resilience in the very vulnerabilities they once feared.

## Self-Perception Challenges

As men grapple with a decline in sexual desire, they often face a crucial barrier that's closer to home than they might think—self-perception. How you see yourself can significantly influence every facet of your life, including your libido. Sometimes, the internal dialogue we engage in can be our own worst enemy. Self-perception challenges aren't just about physical appearance or attractiveness; they extend into competence, self-worth, and how we envision our roles in relationships.

These challenges may begin subtly and, over time, amplify into formidable obstacles. For some, it starts with a single moment of doubt. Perhaps it's a fleeting thought of inadequacy that quickly grows as stressors accumulate. This internal narrative influences outward behaviour, often perpetuating a cycle of avoidance and withdrawal. Men might find themselves shying away from intimacy and vulnerability, creating a chasm where there should be connection and desire.

Understanding the root of these negative self-perceptions is imperative. Often, these challenges stem from unrealistic societal expectations. Men are bombarded with messages about how they should look, perform, and express themselves. The idealistic portrayals in media can distort our understanding of masculinity and virility, embedding ideas that success and desirability are conditional on superficial traits and performance metrics. This creates a dissonance that can quickly erode self-esteem.

Addressing these self-perception challenges requires deliberate introspection. Begin by identifying the triggers that amplify negative thoughts. Are these thoughts related to past experiences, media consumption, or criticisms internalised over time? Recognising these patterns is the first step in challenging the destructive narrative you've built around your self-worth and masculinity. More critically, it's about reframing these narratives and embracing a broader, more inclusive understanding of what it means to be desirable and competent.

An essential aspect of overcoming self-perception barriers is cultivating self-compassion. Consider how you speak to yourself versus how you might comfort a close friend. Why is it easier to extend kindness outward than inward? Practising self-compassion entails accepting that imperfections and vulnerabilities don't diminish your worth. In fact, they can enrich your relationships, building a more authentic and profound connection with your partner. It's about embracing the fullness of who you are without judgment.

Developing a positive self-view isn't an overnight transformation. It's a journey that involves reconstructing deeply held beliefs and being open to different perspectives. Engage in activities that enhance your self-awareness, whether it's through mindfulness practices, journaling, or therapeutic sessions. These methods provide space to explore aspects of yourself that perhaps you've avoided or overshadowed. They can reintroduce you to parts of your identity that you've unjustly criticised or ignored.

Moreover, it's essential to view perceived failures or setbacks not as confirmations of inadequacy but as opportunities for growth and new learning experiences. Every challenge faced can deepen your understanding of yourself, equipping you with insights geared towards personal and relationship improvement. Reframe setbacks as pivotal moments that propel you forward rather than hold you back. Over time, this resilience builds a more robust self-image, grounded in authenticity and confidence.

Engage openly with your partner about these perceptions. In doing so, you create an environment of trust and understanding, where dialogue can thrive without fear of judgment or rejection. Your partner can provide support, reassurance, and a perspective that you might find difficult to see yourself. This shared journey can strengthen your bond and foster an environment where your libido can naturally flourish. Honesty and vulnerability aren't just therapeutic; they're attractive and vital to rekindling intimacy.

Ultimately, reshaping your self-perception involves aligning more closely with what truly matters to you, free from the shackles of external validation. It emphasizes a holistic appreciation of self that intertwines physical, emotional, and intellectual facets of your being. By acknowledging and actively working through self-perception challenges, you equip yourself with a new perspective, one that fuels your libido and enriches your relationship. All this leads to a more satisfying and liberated intimate life.

## Addressing Misconceptions

In the maze of cultural narratives about male libido, misconceptions lurk like minotaurs, often steering men away from understanding their own sexual desires and functioning. These misunderstandings can cloud the truth about libido loss and bolster feelings of inadequacy or failure. Addressing them head-on is not just about dispelling myths, but also about fostering a healthier dialogue about male sexuality.

One of the most persistent misconceptions is the perception that a man's interest in sex is unchanging and perpetual. Society tends to portray male libido as a constant that should burn with the intensity of a thousand suns from adolescence until the twilight years. However, the reality is strikingly different. Libido naturally waxes and wanes influenced by myriad factors. Recognising that these changes are normal and do not indicate a lack of masculinity is crucial in overcoming self-imposed barriers.

There's also the misleading belief that libido is purely driven by physical needs, a mechanical impulse divorced from emotional or psychological states. Many men grow up thinking that sexuality is purely physical, but this overlooks how stress, emotional health, and relational dynamics interweave to affect desire. The interplay of mind and body cannot be undermined. It's fundamental to acknowledge that our mental state is deeply tied to our sexual well-being and addressing mental health is as essential as physical health in maintaining libido.

Adding to these misconceptions is the notion that libido decline is an inevitable consequence of ageing. While hormonal changes can impact libido, they don't spell the end of a fulfilling sexual life. Understanding that age-related decline can be managed or even prevented with appropriate lifestyle changes and medical interventions is empowering. Highlighting stories of vibrant sexual relationships into later life can inspire a more balanced perspective.

Miscommunications about libido aren't limited to murmurs among the uninformed; they extend to medical advice. Some men hesitate to seek help when they notice a drop in their sexual desire, fearing they'll be prescribed medication regardless of their personal context. While pharmaceuticals can play a role, especially in cases of hormonal imbalances, there are also numerous natural and lifestyle interventions to consider first. Seeking help from healthcare professionals who advocate for a holistic approach can ensure that all potential causes are addressed, including psychological and relational factors.

The stigma associated with discussing libido can inhibit open communication. Many feel ashamed to express their vulnerabilities about their sexual desires. This can lead to further misunderstandings within relationships. Partners may wrongly interpret a decline in libido as a sign of infidelity or lack of attraction. Establishing an open dialogue with partners where honest discussions about desires, fears, and even medical conditions can occur without judgement is essential for mutual understanding and support.

Another damaging misconception is the belief that libido decline is exclusively a male problem. In truth, sexual desire is a dynamic dance between partners and can be affected by both parties' physical and emotional states. Exploring the female perspective and understanding that she too may be facing her own challenges can lead to more compassionate interactions and collaborative problem-solving.

A pervasive myth is that loss of libido means a loss of love. This conflation can be damaging, causing significant strain on relationships. It's important to disentangle love from sexual desire, understanding that they can still coexist independently while working towards rekindling the passion. A temporary dip in libido doesn't reflect the depth of feeling but can usher an opportunity to deepen intimacy in non-sexual ways.

Importantly, many men believe that they must conquer this challenge alone, often isolating themselves due to feelings of shame or inadequacy. This is far from the truth. Reaching out for support, whether it's from loved ones, professionals, or peer groups, can provide perspective, encouragement, and practical strategies for overcoming libido-related challenges. Community and connection can be crucial allies in the journey towards restoring desire.

By dismantling these misconceptions, men can pave the way for a deeper understanding of their sexual health, free from stereotypes and stigmas. This clarity allows for a more nuanced and empowering approach to libido loss, moving from a sense of failure to one of potential and growth. The path to overcoming these barriers isn't just about reigniting desire; it's about reclaiming agency over one's sexuality and fostering more authentic and fulfilling relationships.

# Chapter 13:
## Enhancing Sexual Confidence

Building sexual confidence is about nurturing a profound belief in oneself, allowing you to embrace your desires and communicate openly with your partner. The journey begins with fostering self-esteem, which acts as the foundation for a positive body image and self-acceptance. By acknowledging your unique attributes and letting go of unhealthy comparisons, you can shift your perception towards one of appreciation and pride. Techniques such as visualization and affirmations can further enhance confidence, empowering you to navigate intimacy with authenticity and ease. As you cultivate this confidence, it naturally translates into more fulfilling and passionate experiences, creating a ripple effect that strengthens both your sense of self and your relationship. As we move forward, these strategies will provide the groundwork for a more enriched, connected partnership, offering a renewed sense of intimacy and pleasure.

## Building Self-Esteem

Self-esteem is the cornerstone of sexual confidence. A well-rounded sense of self-worth not only impacts your emotional and psychological health but plays a vital role in how you perceive and engage with your partner intimately. Building self-esteem isn't just about feeling good in a general sense. It's about dismantling the barriers that prevent you from enjoying a fulfilling, confident sexual life. Sexual confidence thrives when you are content and assured in who you are, intricately linked with your self-perception.

The first step to enhancing self-esteem involves self-awareness. How do you see yourself? Are you overly critical in areas where you could practise self-compassion instead? Start by recognising your strengths and accomplishments. Write them down. It can be as simple as remembering times when you've felt strong and capable or when you've handled a challenging situation with grace. These reflections will pave the path towards recognising your value beyond superficial attributes.

Physical appearance often plays a significant role in how men perceive their self-worth. However, it's important to expand this view and focus not just on outer attributes but also on the qualities that cannot be measured by the eye. Focus on what makes you an incredible partner, whether it's your kindness, intelligence, or humour. By shifting this focus, you empower yourself with an image that transcends physicality and roots firmly in authenticity.

Building self-esteem is also about stepping outside of your comfort zone. Engaging in new activities or hobbies can foster a sense of achievement that bolsters your confidence. Try setting small, achievable goals that align with your interests. As you accomplish these goals, they build a bank of positive experiences and successes that reinforce your internal narrative, your sense of what you can achieve, and who you ultimately are.

Relationships play an undeniably powerful role in enhancing self-esteem. A supportive partner who appreciates you for who you are can have a transformative impact on how you see yourself. This isn't just about receiving validation; it's about being in an environment where mutual encouragement thrives. Celebrate each other's joys and share in challenges, which builds relational strength and fosters self-assurance.

Equally important is learning to set boundaries and communicate them effectively. This is crucial in retaining your self-esteem and avoiding a situation where you feel overwhelmed or insecure. Practise saying "no" when necessary, and don't be afraid to express what makes you uncomfortable. Remember, safeguarding your own comfort is not selfish; it's a vital part of maintaining your emotional health and self-confidence.

Mindfulness is another tool that can aid in building self-esteem. By being present, you can shed judgments and see situations for what they truly are, rather than what your insecurities might craft. Practising mindfulness involves focusing on the here and now, observing thoughts and feelings without criticism. Through this practice, you develop deeper insights into self-awareness and cultivate an appreciation for who you are, not who you think you should be.

It's equally vital to challenge negative self-beliefs that erode self-esteem. These beliefs often manifest in critical inner dialogues, such as thinking you're "not enough" or that past failures define you. Start by paying attention to these thoughts. Then, counter them with positive affirmations and evidence of past successes. Over time, this shift can transform your inner narrative, empowering you to see yourself in a more positive light.

Professional support can be immensely beneficial for those who find it difficult to build self-esteem on their own. Therapy or counselling provides a safe space to explore deeper issues that may be affecting your self-perception. A professional can guide you through exercises and offer tools that help reinforce a positive self-view, which in return, enhances your sexual confidence.

Building self-esteem is an ongoing journey, one that requires patience and commitment. Practise self-compassion, acknowledging that setbacks are a natural part of the process. Every small victory over insecurity deserves recognition. Over time, these build into significant strides toward a healthier self-image.

Finally, remember that self-esteem is not about perfection but about embracing your true self, with all your strengths and imperfections. This genuine acceptance not only enhances your personal life but deeply enriches your sexual confidence, allowing you to engage with your partner more openly and passionately. By building a robust sense of self-worth, you create a foundation where sexual confidence can thrive, leading to more intimate, satisfying relationships.

## Positive Body Image

When it comes to enhancing sexual confidence, one often overlooked component is the power of a positive body image. How we view our bodies can significantly influence our level of comfort in intimate situations. A positive body image isn't simply about how others view us, but rather how we perceive ourselves. Your perception sets the stage for your sexual confidence, impacting interactions with your partner and your own self-esteem.

It's crucial to acknowledge that developing a positive body image doesn't mean aspiring to unrealistic ideals often portrayed in media. Rather, it involves embracing your unique physical self. Recognizing the diverse and individual qualities that make you who you are is empowering. It's about shifting the focus from perceived flaws to appreciating the myriad of strengths and capabilities your body possesses.

A positive body image isn't static; it's something that evolves with conscious effort and perspective changes. Incorporating daily practices that promote self-acceptance is pivotal. One effective method is the use of affirmations. Regularly affirming that you are comfortable and happy in your own skin can gradually replace negative narratives that may have lingered for years. Additionally, surrounding yourself with positive influences, whether through friends, family, or media consumption, can reinforce a healthy self-image.

Physical activity is not just beneficial for improving physical health, as discussed in Chapter 5, but also has a significant impact on body image. Engaging in activities that you enjoy can enhance how you perceive your physical self. Whether it's a sport, a workout regimen, or a simple daily walk, these activities increase endorphins and enhance your mood, adding a palpable boost to your self-esteem. You celebrate what your body can do, rather than solely focusing on how it looks.

Furthermore, the role of clothing and personal style shouldn't be underestimated. Dressing in a way that feels authentic and comfortable can drastically affect how you carry yourself. Clothing that fits well and makes you feel confident can serve as a subtle yet powerful tool in fostering a positive body image. It's about feeling comfortable in your own skin, which can extend to feeling more at ease in intimate moments with your partner.

Your partner's perspective can also play a significant role in shaping your body image. A relationship built on mutual respect and admiration can be a safe haven for exploring and enhancing each other's self-image. Open communication, as explored in Chapter 6, facilitates understanding and support. Discussing body insecurities with your partner can demystify concerns and transform them into opportunities for closeness and mutual support.

Of course, dealing with negative body thoughts is a natural part of this journey. It's important to confront these thoughts head-on rather than suppress them. Recognising the triggers and underlying causes for these perceptions, which may be explored in tandem with the psychological contributors identified in Chapter 4, can be insightful.

This awareness allows for the development of personalised coping mechanisms that counteract these negative patterns.

Mindfulness, as covered in Chapter 11, can also be a powerful ally in fostering a positive body image. Mindfulness practices such as meditation and body scanning encourage you to observe your body without judgement. These exercises help cultivate an awareness of the body in space, fostering an acceptance and appreciation of its form and function. Emphasising what your body feels and experiences rather than how it looks can divert focus from superficial to substantial.

In cultivating a positive body image, it's essential to create a supportive environment. Whether it's through joining community groups, seeking professional guidance, or engaging in online forums, sharing experiences with others going through similar journeys can be incredibly validating. It's an opportunity to learn and grow from shared vulnerabilities, ultimately leading to a strengthened sense of self.

It's perfectly normal to have days where self-image feels diminished. Embracing this as part of the human experience, rather than a failure, is a step toward acceptance. Understanding that no one is without insecurities can reframe your perspective and focus on improving your unique relationship with your body. As you nurture this relationship, you'll likely find that it translates to more fulfilling and confident intimate interactions.

The journey towards a positive body image is deeply personal but intertwined with broader elements of self-esteem and confidence, as highlighted in Chapters 12 and 21. Building this foundation is not merely about feeling good naked—it's about feeling whole and confident in all facets of life, creating ripples in your intimate relationship.

Ultimately, a positive body image is not the destination but part of an ongoing life journey. As you continue to work towards accepting and celebrating the body you have, you empower yourself to engage more openly and confidently in your sexual and relational life. This process not only enhances intimacy with partners but is also a profound act of self-love and respect, cultivating a resilient and joyful existence.

## Techniques to Boost Confidence

In the realm of sexual confidence, it's easy to forget that confidence is as much about the mind as it is about the body. Men often find themselves caught in a web of self-doubt, cynicism, and unrealistic expectations that can cloud their minds and dilute their assurance. But the promise of renewed confidence lies within reach, and there are effective techniques to rebuild this crucial facet of intimacy.

One powerful method to enhance confidence is through self-reflection and acknowledging one's own strengths. Men can sometimes be their own harshest critics, overlooking their positive traits and contributions. Engaging in regular introspection, perhaps through journaling or meditative reflection, allows men to identify positive attributes and accomplishments. By focusing on what they do well, rather than fixating on perceived flaws, they begin to see themselves in a new light. This shift in perception can be transformational, empowering individuals to approach intimacy with newfound assurance.

It's also imperative to cultivate a sense of *body positivity*. The media can be relentless in bombarding us with images of "ideal" body types, often leading to diminishing self-esteem. Encouraging men to view their bodies with appreciation rather than critique is essential. Simple practices such as standing naked in front of a mirror and expressing gratitude for the body's capabilities can reinforce confidence. Fitness regimes that focus on strength rather than aesthetics may also help foster a positive connection with one's body.

Furthermore, setting realistic goals in personal and professional life can bolster confidence. When ambitions are grounded in reality and aligned with one's values, the sense of achievement boosts self-esteem—this success in one aspect of life often flows into other areas, including sexual confidence. Realising that perfection isn't attainable, but personal growth is, can alleviate undue pressures to perform flawlessly.

The significance of effective communication cannot be overstated. Talking openly with a partner can open pathways to greater understanding and intimacy. When men feel heard and understood by their partner, it nurtures a secure environment where genuine confidence can flourish. Initiating candid discussions about desires, fears, or any insecurities ensures mutual support, paving the way for deeper connections.

Visualisation is another technique that can enhance confidence. Imagining successful sexual scenarios can prepare the mind for real-life encounters, transforming anxiety into anticipation. Creating a mental picture where one feels confident, connected, and in control can be mentally rehearsed to instil a sense of competence when the time comes.

Mindfulness practices are instrumental as they tether the mind to the present moment, steering it away from anxiety about past failures or future pressures. Techniques like mindful breathing, grounding exercises, or even progressive muscle relaxation can reduce stress, clear the mind, and centre attention on the experiences of now. By anchoring oneself in the present, one can engage with their partner without distraction or apprehension, enhancing both confidence and connectivity.

For some, engaging with professional services such as counselling or sex therapy might be beneficial. Such services provide safe spaces to address deep-seated anxieties or misconceptions surrounding sexual performance. Professional guidance offers tailored strategies that cater to individual needs, leading to a stronger and more confident sexual presence.

Moreover, embracing vulnerability can paradoxically lead to greater self-assuredness. When men allow their partners to witness their insecurities and struggles, they dismantle walls that inhibit authentic connection. This transparency fosters trust and intimacy, turning perceived weaknesses into strengths. Allowing oneself to slip occasionally without punishment encourages resilience and endurance.

Lastly, don't underestimate the simple but profound impact of a balanced lifestyle on confidence. Regular exercise, a nutritious diet, ample sleep, and moderated substance use build a foundation not just for physical health but also for mental resilience. When the body and mind are well-nurtured, sexual confidence naturally finds firm footing.

The journey to enhancing sexual confidence is deeply personal, steeped in self-discovery and growth. Through a combination of realistic goal setting, effective communication, positive self-perception, and mindfulness, men can rebuild and reinforce the confidence that is integral to intimate relationships. Each step towards confidence sets the stage for richer, more fulfilling experiences in the bedroom, reigniting passion and strengthening the bonds of intimacy.

# Chapter 14:
## Rediscovering Sensuality

In the transformative journey of reigniting a dwindling flame of desire, rediscovering sensuality emerges as a vital chapter. It's about being acutely awake to the language of touch and the subtleties of physical sensation. Realigning with the experiential world, partners can unveil layers of dormant pleasures, embarking on a quest to foster deeper, more meaningful connections. By focusing on these personal explorations, lovers can transcend mere functionality, discovering new terrains of pleasure and turning mundane interactions into a symphony of delight. This chapter invites you to embrace a dual voyage: one of personal awakening and shared discovery with your partner, crafting a canvas where intimacy flourishes and the essence of sensuality revitalises the core of your relationship. Through mindful attention and openness to new experiences, the essence of passionate living can be reclaimed, reinforcing the vibrant tapestry of intimacy daily.

### Tuning into Physical Sensations

Rediscovering sensuality begins with immersing oneself in the tapestry of physical sensations. Sensuality is often misinterpreted as solely sexual, yet, at its essence, it's about fully experiencing the moment with all the senses tuned to their peak. Whether through touch, taste, sight, sound, or smell, our bodies are capable of providing valuable insights that not only enhance intimacy but also enrich our daily lives.

Imagine sitting quietly, the steady beat of your heart gently stirring beneath your chest. Tuning into this rhythm can be a powerful first step in awakening sensual awareness. Many of us rush through life, barely noticing the simple joys and sensations our bodies experience. The soft breeze against your skin, the warmth of the sun on your face, or the soothing cadence of your breath all serve as natural gateways into a deeper understanding of yourself and your desires.

Understanding these sensations starts with mindfulness, which many find challenging in today's fast-paced world. But devoting time to explore what your body tells you is invaluable. Begin with small steps: a deliberate focus on the tactile sensations of washing your hands or the subtle flavours in your morning tea. This guided attention can gradually extend into your intimate relationships, transforming the way you connect with your partner.

The sense of touch holds a special place in intimacy. It's not just about sexual touch but the myriad of ways two bodies can communicate. A gentle caress, a knowing squeeze of the hand, or a lingering hug can say more than words ever could. Physical connection helps to relieve stress, release endorphins, and foster a sense of belonging, contributing to an open and sensual mindset.

Harnessing the power of sound can also enhance sensual experiences. Music, the natural symphony of the outdoors, or even the gentle voice of a loved one can evoke emotional responses that deepen your connection to the moment. Consider creating a playlist of songs that make you feel alive, sensual, or relaxed. Listening to these tracks with your partner can create shared experiences, enhancing emotional and physical intimacy.

Our sense of smell, forever intertwined with memory and emotion, can transport us instantly to other times and places. This can be harnessed sensually to create a bonding atmosphere. The aroma of a loved one's cologne or the scent of fresh linen can evoke strong emotional responses and contribute to a tactile setting that encourages relaxation and intimacy.

However, achieving full sensual engagement often requires overcoming some barriers. Cultural influences and personal beliefs might have taught us to be wary of bodily pleasures or distrusting of our senses. Recognising these limitations is the first step toward breaking free from them. Encourage yourself to explore the physical sensations associated with freedom and pleasure, embracing them as a fundamental part of your life.

It's important for you and your partner to communicate openly about what you both find pleasurable. Experimenting with different forms of touch and finding new ways to engage all five senses can add layers to your physical connection. This doesn't have to be a chore; rather, it can be a playful exploration that shares mutual benefits and grows your relationship.

Even the art of eating can play a role in rediscovering your sensual self. Engaging with food on a sensory level—savouring each bite, indulging in various textures and tastes—not only can provide pleasure but also foster a greater appreciation for bodily sensations. Try cooking together, engage in a tasting adventure, and enjoy the bonding experience it provides.

It's worth noting that getting in tune with your physical sensations requires patience and practice. Don't be discouraged if immediate results aren't apparent. Instead, approach this journey with curiosity and an open mind. Each small step forward matters and contributes to a larger transformation of enhancing your sensual awareness.

Finally, remember that rediscovering sensuality isn't just about reigniting physical intimacy but also about gaining a deeper insight into your own bodily experience. By fully engaging with our senses, we can enrich our intimate lives and grow closer to those we love.

Through this journey of exploration, passion can blossom anew, creating a symphony of sensations that resonate with both partners, fostering a profound and enduring connection.

## Enhancing Sensual Experiences

Rediscovering sensuality isn't just about reigniting a lost flame; it's about exploring the intricate dance of touch, emotion, and connection that can significantly deepen intimacy in a relationship. It offers a journey back to the basics, where pleasure isn't merely a goal but a lived experience, a reminder of the profound ease and simplicity that can be found in mutual enjoyment. Sensual experiences involve more than just physical touch; they represent an embracing of vulnerability, trust, and the many ways in which we can show love and desire for our partners. This return to sensuality is about expanding the realms of what it means to be intimate, to be close, and to be in harmony with both oneself and another.

To begin this exploration of sensuality, one must first tune into the physical sensations that define our bodies' interactions with the world. This attunement requires a shift in focus, from chasing the climactic and often elusive 'big moment' to savouring each sensation as it happens. By embracing the feel of a soft gust of wind, the warmth of a loved one's skin, or the subtle scent of their presence, partners learn to appreciate the multifaceted nature of touch. Awareness becomes the key that unlocks new levels of intimacy, allowing even the smallest encounters to become meaningful and profound.

Incorporating mindfulness into sensuality encourages a deeper connection with one's own body and desires. By practising mindfulness, couples can enhance their experiences by being present, attentively listening to each other's needs, and avoiding distractions that detract from the moment. This focus helps redefine what touch can mean in a relationship, developing a shared language of gestures and caresses that are intimately tailored to each other's likes and dislikes. Such attentiveness not only improves physical connection but fosters an emotional and psychological closeness that strengthens the partnership's core.

Exploring new avenues of pleasure opens the door to enhanced sensual experiences. It's about finding delight and thrill beyond the standard confines of intimacy. This exploration might involve trying out different textures, temperatures, or even a rearrangement of the environment. The key is not to seek novelty for novelty's sake but to identify what brings joy and stimulates the senses in a fulfilling way. Simple additions—a breeze of essential oils, softer fabrics, or dimmed lighting—can transform a routine encounter into a tapestry of sensations, each layer contributing to a richer, more immersive experience.

Communication plays an indispensable role in this process, as partners need to express and understand each other's evolving desires. Open, honest dialogue about what is enjoyable or what could be improved creates a foundation of trust. Couples are encouraged to discuss their preferences and boundaries, fostering a non-judgmental space where suggestions are welcomed and change is both an adventure and a shared pursuit. In these conversations, empathy reigns supreme, ensuring that both partners feel heard and valued.

Adding to the realm of verbal communication is the language of nonverbal cues—those subtle messages that our bodies convey without words. These could be in the form of eye contact, the pace of breathing, or the gentle squeeze of a hand. Reading these signals effectively can deepen the mutual understanding of each other's needs intensively. It's a reminder that sometimes, the most eloquent expressions of love and desire come not through spoken word but through a gaze, a touch, or the silent understanding shared between two people.

Sensuality isn't restricted to the bedroom. It thrives in shared experiences that connect couples outside traditional settings, weaving intimacy into the fabric of everyday life. This could manifest through activities like cooking together, dancing, or even a simple walk holding hands. Such moments cultivate an environment of continuous closeness and shared joy, reinforcing the bond in a myriad of small, yet powerful ways. The goal here is to maintain a continuous flow of connection that sustains passion and intimacy in daily interactions.

Furthermore, rediscovering and enhancing sensuality can help dismantle societal and personal misconceptions about intimacy that frequently burden men. For some, there's an unspoken pressure to perform, proving virility rather than relishing the softer, slower, deeply rewarding aspects of closeness. By focusing on sensuality, men not only challenge these preconceived notions but also find themselves enjoying deeper satisfaction and connection that weren't previously imagined.

Lastly, the pursuit of enhanced sensual experiences invites couples into a space of playful exploration, encouraging them to be curious and adventurous. This aspect of relationship-building is crucial—it invites humour, spontaneity, and a lightheartedness that can alleviate the serious tones intimacy often assumes under stress. Whether it's by stepping out of comfort zones with new positions or simply laughing together during an awkward moment, these experiences enrich the emotional tapestry of the relationship.

In conclusion, enhancing sensual experiences is a dynamic process that requires intention, exploration, and communication. It's a reminder to cherish the art of touch and the simplicity of shared moments. Such a journey not only revitalises physical connection but also fosters profound emotional ties. By gradually embracing these practices, partners can strengthen their bond and rediscover the joy and fulfilment that deep sensuality can bring to their intimate lives.

## Exploring New Avenues of Pleasure

As we delve deeper into rediscovering sensuality, it becomes essential to explore new avenues of pleasure. In the realm of intimacy, novelty can often be the key to unlocking doors that have gradually closed over time. Relationships can sometimes fall into patterns that might inadvertently dull the senses, making it crucial to inject fresh experiences and sensations into your intimate life. Variety doesn't just spark curiosity; it redefines your shared sensual journey, reminding you of the deep bond and pleasure that lie at the core of your relationship.

Exploring new avenues of pleasure begins with a willingness to communicate your desires and fantasies openly. Discussing what arouses, intrigues, or excites you can be invigorating, allowing you and your partner to embark on a shared adventure. Open dialogue ensures that both partners feel heard and valued, fostering an environment where exploration feels safe and exciting rather than intimidating. Remember, these conversations don't need to transpire all at once; they can evolve naturally, revealing layers of preferences and curiosities over time.

Part of this exploration involves breaking free from the constraints of routine. Routine can be comforting but can also become a barrier to spontaneity and new experiences. Consider experimenting with different times of the day for intimacy, or explore new settings that might inspire a sense of excitement. A change in scenery—whether it's a romantic getaway or simply a different room in the house—can rekindle interest and passion, offering a fresh perspective on familiar experiences.

Touch, a fundamental aspect of sensuality, is another powerful area for exploration. The human body is sensitive to myriad sensations, which can transform the way you perceive touch. Take time to discover which textures, temperatures, and pressures evoke the most powerful responses in both you and your partner. Paying attention to these details transforms touch from a routine gesture into a profound, connecting experience. Gentle, exploring touches can turn into more intense sensations, with subtle variations enhancing mutual pleasure.

Engaging the senses beyond touch can profoundly affect your sexual experiences. Listening to music can create an emotional backdrop, setting the tone and pace for an intimate encounter. Scent, too, plays a critical role in building anticipation and arousal. Choosing fragrances that evoke pleasant memories or exciting new ones can enhance the mood. Similarly, taste can be integrated into your explorations—sharing a favourite food or drink could become part of a sensual ritual, enhancing connection through shared enjoyment.

Engagement of these senses ensures that intimacy becomes a full-bodied experience, where every moment is charged with meaning and pleasure. While exploring pleasure, it's valuable to acknowledge that comfort zones will differ between partners. One partner might be eager to try, while the other prefers to take things slower, which is perfectly normal. Mutual respect and patience are key; take baby steps together and ensure each exploration is consensual and joyful.

Modern technology can also serve as a tool for exploration in a relationship, offering a variety of intimate aids and resources. Whether it's reading couples' guides together or exploring items designed to enhance pleasure in safe and consensual ways, technology can open avenues that might not have been accessible before. Approaching these with curiosity rather than apprehension can enrich the shared experience, fostering an understanding of each other's intricate desires and boundaries.

Language, too, can be explored as a pathway to pleasure. Speaking affirmations or fantasies out loud can be incredibly freeing and empowering. Words hold power and can influence mood, arousal, and connection. Reciting poetry or simply engaging in pillow talk encourages a deeper, more intimate connection. The exchange of soft words or shared humour can act as a bridge, closing the gap between daily life and moments of intimacy.

Keep in mind that exploring new avenues doesn't solely revolve around physical aspects. Emotional depth plays an equally vital role in sensuality. Prioritising emotional intimacy—through acts of kindness, empathy, and understanding—creates a solid foundation upon which physical exploration can thrive. The stronger the emotional bond, the freer both partners will feel to express their desires fully. Emotional closeness reinforces the trust needed to venture into new territories of sensuality, making each experience a shared achievement.

It's important to emphasise that there is no single right path when exploring new avenues of pleasure; what works for others may not suit every couple. The journey is deeply personal, calling for a tailored approach. Be open to trial and error, and regard each discovery, whether it's a triumph or a learning experience, as valuable. This exploration doesn't have to be hurried—taking the time to understand what speaks to both partners most deeply ensures lasting benefits.

Lastly, set aside time to reflect on each experience together. This reflection can be just as fulfilling as the exploration itself, fostering continued joy and openness in the relationship. Engaging in candid conversations about what felt good or what could be adjusted keeps the channels of communication open and the partnership dynamic and responsive to each other's evolving desires.

In the grand tapestry of rediscovering sensuality, exploring new avenues of pleasure is a vibrant thread that adds colour and depth. It requires effort, openness, and sometimes courage, but the rewards—a revitalised sense of connection, deeper intimacy, and a renewed zest for shared exploration—are immeasurable. The journey itself, filled with moments of discovery and joy, becomes a testament to the resilience and creativity of a partnership committed to growth and closeness.

# Chapter 15:
# Exploring Sexual Health and Wellness

Embarking on the journey of sexual health and wellness is vital for reigniting passion and enhancing intimacy in your relationship. It's more than just maintaining physical health; it's about understanding and nurturing every aspect of your sexual well-being. Regular health check-ups are fundamental, serving as proactive measures to ensure both partners can enjoy a fulfilling sexual relationship without the worries of underlying health concerns. Awareness and prevention of sexually transmitted infections (STIs) not only safeguard your health but also enhance trust and openness within the relationship. An appreciation of male physiology's intricacies deepens your understanding of what might influence libido, paving the way for informed discussions and shared explorations with your partner. Through these steps, you empower yourself with knowledge and confidence, ready to embrace a more vibrant and connected intimate life.

## Regular Health Check-ups

In the journey to explore sexual health and wellness, regular health check-ups play an indispensable role. While it's tempting to overlook routine visits to the doctor, especially when we're feeling fine, these check-ups are crucial for maintaining overall health, including sexual well-being. Regularly consulting with healthcare professionals provides not just a snapshot of our current health status, but also lays the foundation for preventive care. By addressing potential issues before they evolve into significant problems, you're taking a proactive stance towards maintaining vitality and reigniting passion in your relationship.

Health is not a monolithic concept. It's an intricate interplay between the physical, mental, and emotional facets of our lives. Comprehensive health check-ups cater to this complexity by evaluating various dimensions of well-being. When it comes to sexual health, regular screenings can help uncover issues that might otherwise remain hidden, such as hormonal imbalances or undiagnosed chronic conditions. Identifying these issues early on allows for timely interventions that can rehabilitate your libido and enhance your intimate connections.

Often, men may be hesitant to seek regular medical advice for a variety of reasons. For some, it might be a matter of inconvenience; for others, there might be apprehension stemming from fear of uncovering a problem. However, understanding the benefits of regular check-ups can shift this perception. These appointments offer an opportunity to establish a rapport with your healthcare provider, transforming these visits into a collaborative effort to optimise your health. It's about taking charge, not just reacting to symptoms or ailments when they manifest.

A vital component of these check-ups is the monitoring of hormonal levels, particularly testosterone. Hormonal imbalances, often subtle, can exert a profound influence on sexual desire and performance. Testosterone plays a pivotal role in male libido; its deficiency can lead to decreased interest in sexual activity. Through regular testing, healthcare providers can track changes in hormone levels and suggest interventions such as lifestyle modifications or supplements to address any starting declines.

Besides hormonal evaluations, these appointments usually encompass assessments of heart health, blood pressure, and cholesterol levels. Cardiovascular health is directly linked to sexual function, as the same blood vessels feeding your heart help facilitate erections. Identifying any cardiovascular concerns early can prevent serious health issues down the road, preserving not only your overall well-being but also enhancing your ability to enjoy fulfilling intimate experiences.

Moreover, regular health check-ups act as a gateway to discussions about any reproductive or sexual health concerns you might have. Whether it be erectile dysfunction, premature ejaculation, or fertility worries, having a trusted healthcare professional to talk to can alleviate anxieties and lead to effective solutions. Being open about these issues can be empowering, breaking down stigma and fostering a proactive approach to sexual health.

Psychological health evaluations are another significant aspect of regular health assessments. Issues like stress, anxiety, and depression can profoundly affect sexual desire and satisfaction. Regular check-ups can involve screenings for these conditions, offering pathways to mental health resources when needed. Addressing these concerns holistically often leads to improvements in both mental well-being and sexual health, underscoring the interconnectedness of body and mind.

In the modern world, where health information is abundant yet sometimes overwhelming, regular check-ups stand as a filter to discern what's necessary and relevant for you. Personalised advice based on your specific health profile can be invaluable in navigating the complexities of maintaining sexual health.

Your health journey doesn't have to be walked alone. By engaging actively with healthcare professionals through regular check-ups, you're enlisting allies committed to your wellness. Their expertise, combined with your proactive stance, forms a powerful strategy to prevent potential issues from derailing your intimate experiences. You're investing in yourself and your relationship.

Ultimately, these check-ups represent a commitment not just to sexual health but to overall longevity and quality of life. They're a reminder that maintaining health is a dynamic process, one that requires attention and care. In embracing regular check-ups, you're taking significant steps towards renewed vitality and passion in your intimate life, honouring not only your personal health but also the health of your relationship.

## STI Awareness and Prevention

Understanding sexual health is a vital part of maintaining overall well-being, and STI awareness is a crucial aspect of this understanding. Sexually transmitted infections (STIs) not only impact physical health but can also significantly influence one's psychological and emotional state, which in turn can affect libido and intimate relationships. Traditionally, discussions about STIs have been shrouded in stigma, but breaking this barrier is essential for fostering a healthier and more open approach to sexual health. Let's explore how awareness and prevention strategies can play an instrumental role in preserving not just your physical health, but also the intimacy in your relationship.

To start, it's important to acknowledge the prevalence of STIs. Many people don't realise how common these infections are. In fact, millions are affected globally each year. Yet, the stigma surrounding STIs often prevents open conversations, leading to misunderstandings and complacency in protection and testing. Changing this narrative starts with education and promoting a proactive approach. Knowing the symptoms, understanding the risks, and knowing when to get tested are the foundations of STI awareness. Knowledge empowers individuals, helping them make informed decisions that protect themselves and their partners.

Prevention is our next logical step. The cornerstone of STI prevention lies in practicing safe sex consistently. This includes the use of condoms and dental dams, which serve as effective barriers, reducing the risk of transmission of infections. However, safe sex isn't just about using protection; it's also about communication and honesty with your partner. Discussing sexual histories and STI testing openly can enhance trust and intimacy, demonstrating care for each other's health. Such conversations may initially be uncomfortable, but they are pivotal in building a secure and mutually respectful relationship.

Another key component of prevention is regular health check-ups and screening. Regular STI testing is an essential part of sexual health, especially for those with multiple partners or new sexual relationships. It's important to note that many STIs can be asymptomatic, meaning you may not experience any symptoms but can still transmit the infection. Early detection through testing can lead to better health outcomes and prevent potential complications. Taking charge of your health through regular screenings shows responsibility and commitment to maintaining a healthy relationship with both yourself and your partner.

Vaccination also plays a significant role in STI prevention. Vaccines are available for certain STIs, such as HPV and hepatitis B, which can prevent infection and subsequent health complications. Discussing vaccination options with your healthcare provider can add an additional layer of protection and peace of mind.

The inclusivity of education in STI awareness is crucial. This means integrating diverse sexual orientations, genders, and cultures into educational materials and healthcare discussions. Every individual deserves access to comprehensive sexual health information tailored to their specific needs and lifestyle. By fostering an inclusive dialogue, we promote a more holistic understanding of sexual health that resonates with all aspects of society, broadening the reach and impact of STI awareness and prevention efforts.

Despite best efforts, misunderstandings and misconceptions about STIs and their prevention still linger. One common misconception is the belief that STIs only affect certain demographics. In reality, anyone who is sexually active can contract an STI, making it essential for everyone to be informed and cautious. Moreover, there's often confusion between STIs and other health issues, leading to misdiagnoses or untreated conditions. Educating oneself ensures that the right preventative measures are carried out.

Furthermore, the emotional burden of dealing with an STI can be overwhelming. It's not just the physical impact that one should consider; the emotional and psychological distress can be equally significant. Feelings of shame, guilt, and anxiety are common among individuals diagnosed with an STI. Addressing these emotional repercussions is vital for overall recovery. Having a supportive partner or access to counselling services can greatly help in navigating this challenging time, ensuring that mental health is prioritised alongside physical health.

It's during these times that the strength of an intimate relationship is truly tested. Partners who can provide support and understanding during such challenges often find that their relationships deepen and grow stronger. Open discussions about STI testing, results, and treatment should be approached with compassion and sensitivity. Reinforce mutual support and continuity in your connection, focusing on solutions and strengthening your bond.

Let's not forget the role of technology in STI awareness and prevention. With the rise of telehealth and mobile apps dedicated to sexual health, gaining access to information and services has become more convenient. Features like anonymous consultations, reminders for tests, and educational resources are easily accessible, breaking geographical and social barriers. These modern tools complement traditional healthcare services, increasing outreach and effectiveness in STI prevention strategies.

In conclusion, STI awareness and prevention are integral to both individual health and the health of a relationship. By educating yourself, practicing safe sex, undergoing regular health screenings, and embracing open communication with your partner, you reinforce your commitment to wellness. This proactive approach not only protects your physical health but also nurtures a deeper level of trust and intimacy with your partner, which is crucial for reigniting passion and overcoming challenges related to libido loss. Embrace knowledge and remove the stigma, crafting a healthier, more informed pathway to sexual health and wellness.

## Understanding Male Physiology

The intricate workings of the male body play a crucial role in sexual health and wellness. At the core, male physiology is a sophisticated interplay of organs, hormones, and biological systems designed to facilitate not only reproduction but also pleasure and emotional bonding. Understanding these mechanisms provides a profound comprehension of how disruptions in physiology can lead to challenges in sexual wellness.

The male reproductive system, vital for reproduction and hormone production, comprises key organs like the testes, prostate gland, and penis, each integral to maintaining libido. The testes are particularly significant, producing sperm and crucial hormones like testosterone. This hormone is often described as the lifeblood of male sexual health, influencing everything from physical appearance to sexual desire. Naturally occurring fluctuations in testosterone levels can profoundly impact a man's libido, dictating periods of higher or lower interest in sexual activities.

Importantly, testosterone doesn't operate in isolation. It's part of a complex endocrine system that balances various hormones, each contributing to sexual function. For example, the adrenal glands produce small amounts of testosterone along with cortisol, which plays a significant role in stress response. When stress levels are high, cortisol can increase to the detriment of testosterone production. This hormonal tug-of-war can lead to diminished sexual interest, illustrating how closely linked emotional and physiological health can be.

Beyond hormonal balance, the cardiovascular system is another pivotal component underpinning male physiology. Adequate blood flow is essential for achieving and maintaining erections. The pathway from arousal to erection involves a fascinating series of vascular events. During sexual stimulation, nerve signals lead to the release of chemicals such as nitric oxide that relax blood vessels in the penis, increasing blood flow which engorges the spongy tissues, resulting in an erection. Conditions that impair circulation, such as hypertension or atherosclerosis, can disrupt this process, inhibiting erectile function and, consequently, sexual satisfaction.

Neurologically, the brain is profoundly influential in governing sexual health. Organs and hormones may act as the hardware of male physiology, but the brain serves as the software, interpreting stimuli and working in tandem with the body's physical processes. Neurotransmitters like dopamine and serotonin affect mood and sexual desire, reinforcing the mind-body connection crucial in maintaining a healthy libido. Psychological perception of sexual inputs is also manipulated here, with the brain determining what is, or isn't, arousing.

Age is an inevitable factor that influences male physiology, often bringing a gradual decline in sexual potency and interest. This phenomenon is largely due to the natural decrease in testosterone levels and other age-related changes in body composition, muscle mass, and bone density. While the passage of time alters the physiological landscape of men, it doesn't dictate the end of a vibrant sex life. Understanding these changes engenders a proactive approach to managing them, potentially extending sexual vitality well into older age.

Interestingly, male physiology is also responsive to lifestyle choices. Nutrition, exercise, and habits such as smoking or alcohol consumption considerably impact the body's sexual health. A diet rich in nutrients supports metabolic and hormonal balance, whereas regular physical activity enhances cardiovascular fitness, promoting healthful circulation necessary for sexual function. Conversely, unhealthy habits can lead to conditions like obesity or diabetes, which pose challenges to sustaining a healthy libido.

Moreover, the reproductive system's health isn't just about maintaining sexual activity; it's intricately linked to emotional expressions and relational satisfaction. Male physiology underpins the capacity for emotional connectivity, crucial in intimate relationships. The sensations, emotions, and responses to physical closeness can transcend physical gratification, fostering deeper emotional bonds between partners.

Recognising the signs of physiological imbalances is vital. Fatigue, hair loss, unexplained weight changes, and mood swings might hint at hormonal disturbances. Early intervention can mitigate prolonged sexual health issues, promoting overall well-being. It's pivotal to consult health professionals about any concerns regarding hormonal or physical health to maintain an optimum state of sexual wellness.

Ultimately, an informed understanding of male physiology provides a powerful foundation to restore and sustain sexual health. By acknowledging the factors influencing physiological processes, men can harness this knowledge to overcome obstacles, reignite passion, and foster fulfilling intimate relationships. It's an enlightening journey, transforming challenges into opportunities for growth and renewed connections.

# Chapter 16:
# The Role of Therapy and Counselling

In the journey towards reigniting passion and restoring intimacy, therapy and counselling prove to be invaluable allies, providing a structured space where men and their partners can explore the complexities of libido loss. Engaging with professional guidance helps individuals peel back the layers of emotional and psychological barriers that might hinder sexual desire. Individual therapy empowers men to delve into personal challenges, building a deeper understanding of themselves and enhancing self-esteem. Meanwhile, couples counselling opens up lines of communication, fostering empathy and strengthening the relationship, as both partners work towards a shared goal of emotional and physical closeness. Finding the right therapist, one who appreciates the nuanced challenges faced by men experiencing a decline in sexual desire, is pivotal. The right fit can pave the way for transformative experiences that nurture and sustainably revive the spark in relationships. Through these therapeutic avenues, not only are immediate concerns addressed, but the foundation for a lifelong, fulfilling connection is nurtured.

## Individual Therapy Benefits

Delving into individual therapy can be a transformative experience, especially for men grappling with a decline in sexual desire. There's a unique power in sitting across from a trained therapist and unlocking the mysteries of one's mind and experiences. This process isn't just about talking; it's about discovering who you are beneath layers of societal expectations and personal doubts. Therapy allows for a safe exploration of one's inner world, shedding light on underlying issues that may contribute to a low libido.

Individual therapy offers a space free from judgement, where you can confront personal vulnerabilities that might be affecting your sex drive. Many men live under the pressure of prescribed masculinity, which can perpetuate silence about their struggles. By engaging in therapy, you step away from societal stereotypes and begin a journey that honours your unique experiences and challenges. This process often leads to enhanced self-awareness and an improved sense of identity and confidence, directly impacting your intimate relationships.

For some, therapy becomes a training ground for developing healthier coping mechanisms in response to stressors that typically impact libido. Stress is a notorious libido dampener, but with personalised strategies devised in therapy, you can navigate these challenges more effectively. Learning to manage stress through individual therapy can lead directly to improved sexual desire and overall relationship harmony. Therapists help cultivate resilience, turning stressors into manageable hurdles rather than insurmountable barriers.

Furthermore, therapy aids in unearthing emotional blocks that can obstruct sexual desire. Unresolved issues—whether they're past traumas, current anxieties, or deeply ingrained beliefs—can all contribute to a suppressed libido. Addressing these in individual therapy is akin to lifting a heavy weight from one's shoulders. It clears the mental clutter, allowing for a renewed expression of sexual desire. Each session can bring new insights, ultimately fostering a more fulfilling intimate life.

The therapeutic process also encourages the recognition and dismantling of negative thought patterns. Often, these patterns manifest as self-restrictive beliefs around one's sexual capacity or desirability, exacerbating a cycle of low libido. A therapist can guide you in re-framing these thoughts, helping build a healthier self-perception. This shift alone can be incredibly liberating and can reignite the passion that's been lying dormant.

Security and trust in therapy provide a fertile ground for exploring one's sexual identity beyond the act of sex itself. This exploration can be pivotal for those whose lack of desire is linked to confusion or dissatisfaction with their sexual identity. The therapist serves as a guide, helping navigate this journey of self-discovery, and aiding in reconciling any inner dissensions that inhibit a rewarding sex life.

Therapy's benefits extend beyond individual growth, impacting your relationship dynamics as well. As you evolve personally, you're likely to bring newfound insights and healthy communication strategies back into your partnership, fostering a more supportive and empathetic relationship environment. With your enhanced understanding and communication skills, you're better equipped to articulate your desires and concerns with your partner, laying the groundwork for deeper emotional and physical connection.

Moreover, individual therapy promotes mindfulness, a state of present moment awareness that can significantly enhance your intimate experiences. Mindfulness creates a bridge between the newfound self-awareness gained in therapy and the moment-to-moment experiences with your partner. It allows you to savour each moment without the intrusion of past regrets or future anxieties. This mindful presence can transform not only the depth of your sexual encounters but also enrich everyday interactions with your partner.

Embracing therapy is also about creating a support system. Initially, it might seem daunting to seek help, but engaging with a therapist provides ongoing support, acting as a lifeline during periods of self-doubt or challenge. Through this supportive framework, you're encouraged to take risks, try new approaches, and even stumble along your path towards rekindling your libido. The triumphs and setbacks shared in therapy become stepping stones towards lasting change.

Finally, therapy isn't a quick fix. It demands commitment and openness to introspection. Yet, the rewards it offers are abundant and enduring. Individual therapy can transform your understanding of sexual desire, breaking down not just psychological barriers, but reinforcing those life-enhancing habits that ensure a sustaining and fulfilling intimate relationship. As you venture down this path, you might find that the spark you seek is intricately woven with the person you discover yourself to be.

## Couples Counselling

When it comes to reigniting passion and deepening the connection within a relationship, couples counselling can be an invaluable resource. Often, a decline in sexual desire is not merely an individual's experience but a shared journey between partners. It affects emotional dynamics, mutual satisfaction, and the very fabric of a relationship. That's where counselling steps in, offering a structured environment to explore and address these issues together.

Couples counselling provides a safe space for partners to openly communicate their feelings and concerns. It's not just about addressing the symptoms of libido loss, but delving into underlying issues that might be contributing to it. Many couples find that guided dialogue with a therapist helps them express thoughts they've struggled to articulate, fostering understanding and empathy. This process can unveil unspoken tensions or unmet needs, paving the way for resolutions that reignite desire.

One of the key benefits of couples counselling is the facilitation of better communication. Miscommunication or lack of communication can significantly impact intimacy. In therapy, couples learn effective communication strategies that improve how they connect, discuss, and resolve issues. This doesn't just help with the immediate concerns regarding libido; it builds a stronger, more resilient relationship capable of weathering future challenges.

Therapists often encourage couples to explore the emotional closeness within their relationship. Emotional intimacy is foundational for a fulfilling physical relationship. Through counselling, partners can rebuild trust, address longstanding conflicts, and express vulnerability in a supportive setting. This rebuilding of emotional bridges can lead to a more rewarding physical connection, rejuvenating the bond both in and out of the bedroom.

Moreover, couples counselling assists in joint exploration of solutions. With the guidance of a therapist, partners can collaboratively discover new ways to ignite passion, whether it be through trying new activities, planning dedicated time for intimacy, or redefining what romance looks like in their relationship. This exploratory phase can inject a sense of adventure and novelty into the partnership, helping partners feel more connected and invested in each other.

An often overlooked aspect of couples counselling is its role in addressing external stresses that may compound libido issues. Life's challenges, such as financial strain or parenting responsibilities, can weigh heavily on a relationship. Counselling equips couples with coping strategies to manage external pressures without letting them seep into their intimate life. By placing focus on the relationship's strengths and shared goals, partners can gain a sense of unity and purpose.

Sometimes, couples discover that past experiences or unresolved personal issues are impacting their current relationship. Counselling can be instrumental in helping partners understand these influences and work through them together. Whether it's previous relationship trauma or personal insecurities, unearthing and addressing these aspects within the context of the relationship can lead to healing and strengthened intimacy.

Importantly, couples counselling isn't just about addressing what's wrong. It also highlights what works well within the relationship. Recognising and celebrating the strengths of a partnership can reinforce positive patterns of interaction and bolster the couple's resolve to reignite their connection. Therapists help couples identify and lean into these strengths, reinforcing positive behaviours that support a healthier dynamic.

The decision to attend couples counselling can be intimidating. It requires vulnerability and a willingness to confront uncomfortable truths. However, this act of committing to healing and growth is in itself a powerful step towards transforming the couple's shared journey. For many, it signals a renewed investment in the relationship and a stepping stone towards reigniting desire and building a fulfilling future together.

For men experiencing libido decline, knowing that they aren't alone in the process can be comforting. Couples counselling underscores the notion that relationship issues, including those related to intimacy, are a shared responsibility. Engaging in therapy together ensures that partners walk the path of rediscovery hand in hand, with mutual support and understanding.

As partners move through the counselling process, they gain tools and insights that support ongoing growth and connection. This journey through and beyond counselling can help them not only overcome current hurdles but also prepare them for the complexities of life together, creating a lasting impact on their intimate and emotional lives.

## Finding the Right Therapist

Finding the right therapist can be a transformative journey for men experiencing a decline in sexual desire. Therapy and counselling are not just about addressing immediate concerns but also about fostering a deeper understanding of underlying issues. It's about forging a path towards lasting change and rejuvenated passion. But where does one begin? The first step is identifying what you're looking for in a therapist. It's crucial to find someone whose expertise and approach align with your specific needs and goals.

When selecting a therapist, consider their specialisations. Are they experienced in handling issues related to sexual health, relationships, and personal development? Qualifications are important, but so is the rapport. The therapeutic alliance, or the bond between you and your therapist, is a key predictor of successful outcomes. A strong alliance is built on trust and mutual respect, allowing for open and vulnerable discussions. It's vital to feel safe and understood in this professional space.

Location and logistical concerns might come into play, too. With the convenience of digital technology, many therapists now offer sessions online, which can be a boon for those with hectic schedules or those who might find the traditional face-to-face setting daunting. However, some may prefer in-person interactions for their immediate physical presence and the structured environment they provide. Whatever the format, consistency is key. Regular sessions establish momentum and provide a structured pathway for progress.

The financial aspect is another consideration. Therapy can be a significant investment, so consider what you're able to afford long-term. Some therapists offer sliding scales based on income, and insurance may cover sessions in certain circumstances. Prioritising your mental health should never be seen as an unaffordable luxury but as a critical component of your overall well-being.

Consulting directories and online resources can provide a starting point for finding qualified professionals. Websites often feature therapist profiles, detailing their credentials, areas of expertise, and therapeutic styles. Initial consultations, whether free or at a reduced rate, are an excellent opportunity to gauge compatibility. During this session, pay attention to how comfortable you feel discussing your concerns. Does the therapist listen actively? Are they empathetic?

Beyond credentials, consider the therapeutic approach each professional employs. Some therapists use cognitive behavioural therapy (CBT), which focuses on identifying and changing negative thought patterns. Others may utilise psychodynamic therapy, exploring deep-seated emotional issues from past experiences. Understanding these differences can help you find a therapeutic style that resonates with you.

Another critical factor is the alignment of values and cultural understanding. A therapist who appreciates the nuances of your cultural background or personal identity can provide more personalised support. As men experiencing a decline in sexual desire often battle societal stigmas, having a therapist who can navigate these challenges can be incredibly beneficial.

The journey to finding the right therapist might also involve seeking recommendations. Personal referrals from friends or family members who've had positive experiences can be invaluable. Likewise, some professional organisations provide accreditation and directories of registered therapists, ensuring you have access to reputable practitioners.

Once in therapy, the process requires dedication. Therapy isn't about quick fixes but about building resilience and developing new strategies for addressing life's challenges. A good therapist will help you cultivate self-awareness and equip you with tools to rediscover your desire and enhance relational intimacy.

Remember, it's perfectly acceptable to change therapists if you don't feel the connection you hoped for. Therapy is a personal journey, and it's important for the individual and therapist to be aligned in their objectives. This search is about finding someone who facilitates growth, not someone you settle for due to convenience.

Ultimately, finding the right therapist can empower you to tackle libido loss with renewed vigour. Whether dealing with psychological barriers, confronting lifestyle changes, or navigating complex relationship dynamics, the process offers a collaborative effort. As you embark on this journey, remind yourself that the decision to seek help is a brave and commendable step toward living a more fulfilling life.

With the right therapist, you gain not only a professional ally but someone who guides and supports you as you explore new avenues for rekindling intimacy and passion. As you engage in therapy, you'll learn to view challenges as opportunities for growth, enriching both your personal and relational landscapes in profound and lasting ways.

# Chapter 17:
# Nutrition and Supplements for Libido

Nutrition isn't just about fuelling your body; it's about empowering your vitality and passion. The foods you eat can have a profound effect on your libido, helping to rekindle the fading flames of desire. Embracing a diet rich in nutrients that are known to boost sexual health can inspire a transformative journey. Imagine integrating foods teeming with antioxidants, trace minerals, and vitamins that synergise to optimise hormonal balance and blood flow. Supplements, when chosen wisely and evaluated for efficacy and safety, can act as catalysts, enhancing the natural processes that restore and elevate your sexual drive. With the right nutritional choices, you're not just nourishing your body—you're invigorating your entire being, lighting a path back to the connectivity and intimacy that enrich relationships.

## Foods Known to Boost Libido

In the realm of rekindling passion and enhancing intimate relationships, nutrition can be a key player. What we eat not only fuels our bodies but also plays a significant role in hormonal balance and overall vitality—all crucial factors in maintaining a healthy libido. Let's explore a variety of foods that are known to bolster sexual desire in men, hitting the right notes of taste, nutrition, and libido enhancement.

First on the list is the ubiquitous oyster. Oysters have long been touted as an aphrodisiac, not merely due to folklore but because they're rich in zinc. This mineral is essential for testosterone production, a hormone intimately linked with sex drive. Eating a few oysters might just influence hormonal levels enough to notice a difference in arousal.

If seafood isn't your preference, fear not. Dark leafy greens, like spinach, are another option worth considering. These greens are rich in magnesium, a mineral that boosts blood flow by reducing inflammation and dilating blood vessels. Improved circulation results in the potential for better arousal and erectile function.

Let's not forget about sweet delights like apples and strawberries. While they may not announce themselves as libido enhancers, they're rich in antioxidants such as quercetin. Quercetin can improve circulation and stamina, making these fruits a deliciously discreet addition to your diet for enhancing sexual function.

Meandering over to the spicy side, chilli peppers can enliven more than just your taste buds. Capsaicin, the spicy compound in chillies, triggers the release of endorphins. Endorphins are known mood enhancers, creating a euphoric feeling that can help lower inhibitions and increase sexual desire. Additionally, they promote blood flow—a key element in sexual arousal.

For those with a penchant for sweet indulgences, dark chocolate is a treat that doesn't disappoint. It's loaded with flavonoids and phenylethylamine, an alkaloid known as the 'love chemical'. These compounds stimulate the brain and heighten feelings of attraction, making dark chocolate more than just a dessert but also a passion booster.

Turning our focus to nuts and seeds, we find almonds and walnuts. They're not only convenient snacks but also rich in vital fatty acids. These healthy fats are essential for hormone production and libido maintenance. Including a handful of them in your daily diet could subtly support libido and energy levels.

Olive oil, a staple of the Mediterranean diet, deserves an honourable mention. Rich in monounsaturated fats and vitamin E, olive oil boosts circulation and hormonal balance. This oil can be integrated easily into meals, from drizzling over salads to cooking your favourite dishes. Its benefits extend beyond libido, promoting heart health and overall well-being, which intrinsically support sexual vitality.

Garlic might not be your first choice due to its potent smell, but its benefits can't be ignored. It contains allicin, a compound that enhances blood flow. While you might want some mints on hand, incorporating garlic into your meals can provide long-term benefits to cardiovascular health, indirectly supporting erectile function.

Another interesting contender is the pomegranate. Known as a symbol of fertility, its juice is packed with antioxidants that improve blood circulation and heart health. Regular consumption may lead to increased testosterone levels, bolstering libido in the process.

Lastly, remember the role of hydration in augmenting sexual drive. Watermelon, primarily water, is also high in the amino acid citrulline. This amino acid relaxes blood vessels and enhances blood flow, akin to the effects of some medications used to treat erectile dysfunction, offering a natural and refreshing alternative.

While foods can be instrumental in boosting libido, it's essential to maintain a balanced diet. Over-reliance on any one food might not deliver the desired results. A varied, nutrient-rich diet, supported by comprehensive lifestyle changes including regular exercise and adequate sleep, sets the foundation for sustainable libido enhancement. By incorporating these libido-friendly foods into your daily diet, you're not just nurturing your body, but also paving the way for renewed passion and deeper intimacy in your relationships.

## Importance of Vitamins and Minerals

In the quest to revitalise libido, vitamins and minerals play a pivotal yet often underestimated role. Essential nutrients are the body's building blocks, fuelling countless physiological processes that underpin sexual health. When nutrient intake is inadequate, libido can suffer, along with overall vitality and well-being.

First and foremost, vitamins act as catalysts in the body's biochemistry, supporting hormone balance and neurotransmitter function, both crucial for maintaining a healthy libido. Vitamin D, for instance, is integral not just for bone health but also for hormone production. Low levels of vitamin D have been linked to decreased testosterone, thereby impacting sexual desire in men. Given the prevalence of vitamin D deficiency, especially in regions with limited sunlight, ensuring sufficient intake from dietary supplements or fortified foods is vital.

Another key player is vitamin B complex, a group of vitamins that includes B1 (thiamine), B6 (pyridoxine), and B12 (cobalamin), among others. These vitamins support energy metabolism and are essential for nervous system health. Vitamin B6, in particular, is involved in the synthesis of neurotransmitters such as serotonin and dopamine, which elevate mood and enhance sexual arousal. A deficiency in B vitamins can lead to fatigue and mental sluggishness, diminishing sexual interest and performance.

Minerals are equally significant in this narrative. Zinc, for instance, has long been heralded as a crucial nutrient for male sexual health. Found in high concentrations within the prostate gland, zinc is essential for testosterone production and sperm health. Insufficient zinc intake can lead to lower testosterone levels and decreased libido.

Incorporating zinc-rich foods such as oysters, red meat, and seeds can be beneficial, but supplements might also be considered to ensure optimal levels.

Magnesium is another mineral with multi-faceted roles in libido enhancement. It aids in the relaxation of muscles and the regulation of blood flow, factors important for sexual function. Furthermore, magnesium interacts with chemicals in the brain to reduce stress and promote relaxation, which can alleviate anxieties that inhibit sexual desire. Foods like nuts, leafy greens, and whole grains are excellent sources of magnesium.

Let's not overlook iron, a mineral necessary for maintaining energy levels and reducing fatigue. Iron deficiency, particularly common in young men due to dietary choices, can lead to symptoms like lethargy and weakness, indirectly impacting libido. Ensuring adequate iron intake from lean meats and legumes can counter fatigue, thereby helping maintain interest and stamina in sexual activity.

In addition to these essential nutrients, selenium also deserves a mention. Selenium plays a crucial role in sperm motility and overall reproductive health. Brazil nuts, fish, and eggs are great sources of selenium that can easily be added to a balanced diet.

In the context of libido, these vitamins and minerals are seldom discussed as standalone remedies. Instead, they often contribute to a broader picture of optimal health. A nutrient-rich diet not only supports sexual desire but also boosts confidence, mood, and energy— all of which are critical components in the pursuit of fulfilling relationships.

However, it's important to approach supplementation mindfully. While deficiencies can cause issues, excessive intake, particularly through supplements, can be harmful. Consulting with a healthcare provider ensures that supplementation is necessary and adjusted according to individual needs.

Despite our focus on individual nutrients, it's worth noting that they work synergistically in our bodies. A deficiency or excess in one can affect the balance of others. Thus, a holistic approach to nutrition—embracing a balanced diet packed with varied, whole foods—is often the best strategy for enhancing libido and overall health.

Ultimately, understanding and optimising vitamin and mineral intake forms a crucial step in the journey to rediscovering libido. By fuelling your body with the right mix of essential nutrients, you can set the stage for hormone balance, improved energy levels, and a more vibrant sex life. This approach complements other lifestyle adjustments, medical interventions, and psychological strategies aimed at enhancing sexual health.

Incorporating these nutritional insights into daily practice not only lays the foundation for a robust libido but also fortifies the paths to a healthier, more fulfilling life. By embracing the synergy between physical and nutritional wellness, individuals can unlock a powerful mechanism for reigniting passion and strengthening intimate bonds. The journey to restored desire is intricate, but the roadmap is enriched through mindful attention to vitamins and minerals.

## Evaluating Supplements

Navigating the complex world of supplements can be daunting, especially when it comes to enhancing libido. Men and their partners, already grappling with the intricacies of desire, may feel overwhelmed by the myriad of products promising to reignite passion. However, understanding which supplements are effective and how they work is essential in making informed decisions. This section delves into evaluating the various supplements available, their potential benefits, and considerations for safe use, aiming to provide clarity in your journey towards restoring intimacy.

One of the primary attractions of supplements is their accessibility. Without the need for prescriptions or medical consultations, they offer a direct avenue to potentially boost libido. However, this accessibility necessitates a cautious approach; not all supplements are created equally, and the market is rife with options that range from potentially beneficial to entirely ineffective or even harmful. It's crucial to approach these products with a critical eye and a foundation of knowledge.

Understanding the active ingredients is the first step in assessing a supplement's effectiveness. Common ingredients like L-arginine, maca root, Tribulus terrestris, and ginseng have garnered attention for their potential libido-enhancing properties. Each of these ingredients operates differently in the body, targeting various aspects of sexual health and function. For instance, L-arginine is believed to improve blood flow, which can be beneficial for erectile function, while maca root is often cited for balancing hormones and increasing stamina. When evaluating these ingredients, consider their mechanisms and how they align with your specific needs.

Scientific backing is a crucial component in evaluating supplements. While many options boast traditional and anecdotal evidence, it's vital to prioritise those supported by rigorous scientific studies. Peer-reviewed research provides a more reliable basis for understanding potential benefits and any associated risks. Supplements with strong scientific backing offer more confidence in their use for enhancing libido, ensuring you are not just hoping for an effect but are rather making a choice grounded in evidence.

Dosage and formulation also play significant roles in a supplement's efficacy. It's not just about what ingredients are present but in what quantities and combinations. Some products might offer a blend of several active components, purporting to offer synergistic benefits. When assessing these, consider whether the dosages align with those used in successful studies and if the form of the supplement (e.g., pills, powders, or extracts) is optimal for the body's absorption and use. Often, the effectiveness depends on the precise balance, meaning more isn't always better, and incorrect dosages can lead to diminished effects or side effects.

Safety cannot be overstated when considering supplements for libido. Always scrutinise a product's safety profile alongside its potential benefits. Look for supplements that have undergone third-party testing to ensure quality and purity. Unregulated batches can contain contaminants or substances not listed on the label, posing health risks. It's also wise to consult a healthcare professional before starting any new supplement, as they can advise on possible interactions with medications or pre-existing health conditions, providing an extra layer of security in your libido-enhancing endeavours.

The role of placebo effects should not be overlooked when evaluating supplements. The psychological impact of taking a product with the expectation of increased libido can sometimes result in perceived improvements, irrespective of the actual effectiveness of the supplement. This doesn't diminish the value of potential improvements but highlights the complex interplay between mind and body that can accompany supplement use. Awareness of this effect encourages a balanced perspective, preventing reliance solely on these products while overlooking other crucial factors such as lifestyle adjustments or emotional well-being.

Furthermore, it's important to align supplement use with an overall strategy for enhancing libido, anchored in a healthy lifestyle. Supplements should be seen as complementary to other practices like balanced nutrition, regular physical activity, and establishing emotional intimacy with your partner. A holistic approach amplifies the benefits of supplements, creating an environment where various factors synergise to promote improved sexual health.

Remaining informed and adaptable is fundamental in evaluating and using supplements effectively. Stay abreast of emerging research and be open to adjusting your regimen as needed, allowing for flexibility in response to new insights or changing personal needs. Supplements may offer substantial help, but they are just one of many tools available in your quest to reignite passion.

In sum, evaluating supplements for libido is not just about selecting products that advertise enhanced desire. It's about discerning quality, understanding individual needs, and blending supplementation with broader strategies for sexual health. By grounding your choices in evidence and approaching the process deliberately, you can navigate the supplement landscape with confidence and clarity, ultimately enhancing intimacy and connection in a meaningful and sustainable way.

# Chapter 18:
# Physical Activity and Its Connection to Libido

Physical activity extends far beyond fitness, weaving itself intricately into the fabric of sexual vitality. Engaging in regular exercise isn't just about sculpting the body or improving longevity; it plays a pivotal role in enhancing libido. Studies consistently highlight that men who remain active often experience heightened sexual desire and improved performance. Cardiovascular health, bolstered through activities such as running, swimming, and cycling, directly correlates with sexual function by enhancing blood flow and boosting mood. Endurance, too, is refined through fitness, laying the foundation for sustained intimacy. Exercise also acts as a natural stress reliever, helping to counteract psychological barriers like anxiety and depression that often inhibit libido. This holistic approach, integrating physical health with sexual wellness, not only reignites passion but also fosters a profound connection with one's partner, reaffirming the body's natural zest for a vibrant intimate life.

## Exercises Specifically for Libido

When it comes to enhancing libido, physical activity can be a powerful ally. Exercise is well-known for its myriad of benefits ranging from weight management to mental well-being, but its role in improving sexual desire is particularly significant. The right kind of exercises can boost testosterone levels, improve circulation, and enhance one's self-confidence, all of which are crucial for a robust libido.

First, let's explore strength training. Engaging in regular resistance exercises can significantly increase testosterone levels, a key hormone in male sexual desire. Activities such as weightlifting, push-ups, and squats not only build muscle but also stimulate testosterone production. They're excellent for men of any age, offering a dual benefit of physical fitness and increased sexual energy. Moreover, as you build muscle, you may find your self-image improving, which can further enhance sexual confidence.

Cardiovascular exercises also play a vital role in maintaining a healthy libido. Activities such as running, cycling, and swimming get the heart pumping and improve overall circulation. Improved blood flow is essential for erectile function, which directly impacts sexual performance and satisfaction. Regular cardio workouts help maintain a healthy heart and vascular system, ensuring that all systems are go when the moment arises.

Let's not overlook flexibility and core-strengthening exercises. Incorporating practices like yoga and Pilates into your routine can enhance sexual health by improving flexibility, endurance, and body awareness. These exercises can lead to better performance and satisfaction during intimate moments, as they allow for a greater range of motion and longer-lasting stamina. Additionally, the meditative aspect of yoga can reduce stress levels, further supporting a healthy libido.

Another effective form of workout is High-Intensity Interval Training (HIIT). HIIT sessions involve short bursts of intense exercise followed by recovery periods and are known to boost metabolism and increase energy levels. This type of training can also stimulate the release of growth hormone and testosterone, aiding in muscle growth and sexual health. HIIT is time-efficient and can be adapted to suit personal fitness levels and preferences, making it a versatile option for busy schedules.

It's essential to combine these exercises with regular pelvic floor exercises, often overlooked yet tremendously beneficial. Pelvic floor exercises strengthen the muscles that support sexual organs, leading to improved erectile strength and endurance. Commonly referred to as Kegel exercises, they're discreet and can be performed practically anywhere. To do them, simply contract the muscles you would use to stop urinating. Hold the contraction for a few seconds, then release. Over time, this will improve not only your sexual health but also urinary and bowel function.

Let's not forget the psychological benefits of exercise, which are just as important as the physiological ones. Regular physical activity leads to the release of endorphins, often referred to as the body's natural happiness hormones. The endorphin rush not only enhances mood but can also alleviate stress and anxiety, two common psychological barriers to a healthy libido. When you're more relaxed and in a good mood, your desire naturally follows suit.

The sense of accomplishment that comes from sticking to a regular exercise routine can also do wonders for your self-esteem. When you feel better about yourself and your body, it's likely to reflect positively in your intimate relationships. Confidence can often be a fleeting thing, but physical activity helps fortify it, making it less likely to wane due to common insecurities.

Importantly, it should be noted that extreme exercise or overtraining can have the opposite effect on libido, leading to decreased testosterone levels and fatigue. Balance is key, and listening to your body's signals crucial. Engage in regular, moderate exercise tailored to your body's needs and capabilities to create a sustainable fitness routine that's beneficial to both physical and sexual health.

The journey towards a more fulfilled and vibrant sexual life through exercise is as much about self-exploration as it is about the physical changes you'll experience. Strengthen your body, yes, but also take this opportunity to nurture a healthier relationship with yourself. As you enhance your physical stamina, remember you're also paving the way for improved intimacy and connection with your partner. Exercise is your ally, not just for better health, but for a richer, more satisfying life in all its facets.

## Cardiovascular Health and Sexual Function

We've journeyed through the significance of physical activity in enhancing libido, touching on various aspects that strengthen both body and desire. However, it's essential to highlight the often-underestimated role of cardiovascular health. A healthy heart is not only vital for overall well-being but also intricately linked to sexual function. Understanding this connection can inspire men to take proactive steps towards maintaining robust heart health, ultimately benefiting their intimate lives.

Cardiovascular health plays a pivotal role in sexual function. The heart is responsible for pumping blood throughout our bodies, and adequate blood flow is crucial for a healthy sexual response. When cardiovascular health is compromised, so too is our body's ability to respond to sexual stimuli, which can lead to issues such as erectile dysfunction. Addressing heart health can therefore have a profound and positive impact on sexual performance and satisfaction.

Physical activity is one of the cornerstones of a healthy cardiovascular system. Engaging in regular exercises, especially those that get the heart rate up, like brisk walking, swimming, or cycling, can enhance cardiovascular function. These activities improve blood circulation, reduce blood pressure, and help maintain a healthy weight. All these factors contribute to a healthier heart and ultimately facilitate better sexual performance. Consistent aerobic exercise can also lower the risk of developing chronic conditions that might impede sexual function, such as heart disease or diabetes.

Besides direct physiological benefits, maintaining good cardiovascular health through physical activity can boost confidence levels. Many find that regular exercise helps them feel more energetic and attractive. This uplift in self-esteem can have a direct correlation with sexual desire and performance, as feeling good about oneself can enhance intimacy.

Moreover, good cardiovascular health can relieve stress. Stress is a significant barrier to a healthy libido, as it often leads to anxiety and fatigue, both of which can diminish sexual desire. By engaging in cardiovascular exercise, the body releases endorphins, often referred to as "feel-good" hormones. This natural mood booster can alleviate stress, making room for enhanced sexual desire and more fulfilling intimate experiences.

It's not just about exercise, though. A well-rounded lifestyle that supports cardiovascular health includes a balanced diet. Eating heart-friendly foods like fruits, vegetables, whole grains, and lean proteins can complement the benefits of exercise. These eating habits can help manage cholesterol levels and keep the arteries clear, ensuring that blood flows freely throughout the body, including to the sexual organs.

Hypertension, or high blood pressure, can be a hidden enemy to both cardiovascular and sexual health. High blood pressure damages blood vessels, reducing arterial flexibility and impairing circulation. This condition can silently disrupt the balance needed for a healthy sexual function. Regular cardiovascular activity plays a dual role here: it helps in managing blood pressure levels and protecting your sexual health.

Incorporating mindfulness and relaxation techniques as part of a cardiovascular health plan can also indirectly support sexual function. Techniques like focused breathing, meditation, or yoga can reduce stress levels and improve heart health. These practices encourage a holistic approach to well-being, balancing physical activity with mental and emotional health benefits.

Men often overlook the importance of monitoring their heart health until a problem arises, which can affect sexual health unexpectedly. A proactive stance, involving regular check-ups and understanding risk factors, is invaluable. Many cardiovascular diseases are preventable or manageable with the right lifestyle adjustments. Taking control of heart health can prevent disruptions in sexual function, maintaining not only physical capabilities but also emotional connections with partners.

In conclusion, the nexus between cardiovascular health and sexual function highlights the necessity for focusing on heart health as a means to enhancing libido. It's about creating a cycle of health and vitality where taking care of your heart nourishes your sexual well-being. Adopting regular cardiovascular exercises, a heart-healthy diet, and stress management techniques can, in many ways, clear the path to rejuvenated sexual experiences. This proactive approach isn't just about maintaining physical performance but about nurturing a passionate and intimate relationship that thrives on wellness and vitality.

## The Role of Fitness in Endurance

Understanding the intricate relationship between physical fitness and endurance can offer valuable insights into reigniting sexual desire. Fitness is not merely about building muscles or losing weight; it also involves enhancing endurance, which is pivotal for those looking to bolster their libido.

Endurance is the body's ability to sustain prolonged physical or mental effort. When relating it to sexual activity, it becomes apparent why endurance is crucial. Fitness not only enhances your stamina in everyday tasks but also fuels energy levels necessary for a vibrant sexual life. When we discuss endurance in the context of libido, we are highlighting the capacity for sustained intimate engagement without premature fatigue.

Integrating endurance-based fitness routines can significantly influence blood circulation, a vital component for sexual performance. Regular exercise improves cardiovascular health, which in turn ensures that the heart becomes more efficient at pumping blood. Enhanced blood flow is essential for men, as it directly impacts erectile function. Aerobic activities like cycling, running, or swimming are fantastic for maintaining a healthy heart and boosting overall stamina.

But it's not just about cardiovascular health. Endurance exercise influences hormonal balance in the body. While we know testosterone plays a key role in sexual desire, what's intriguing is how consistent exercise regulates hormones to foster a better mood, reduce stress, and improve sleep. All these aspects are critical as they collectively enhance sexual desire.

Involving yourself in physical activity doesn't have to be a chore. Find something you enjoy, be it brisk walking in the morning, a dance class in the evening, or a weekend hike. The key here is consistency. The more regular the activity, the more pronounced the benefits. Over time, the increased energy levels translate into newfound enthusiasm not just for exercise, but for daily activities, including intimacy. This renewed vigour can result in a noticeable improvement in sexual desire.

Resistance training also has its place in fostering endurance. While often seen as a means to increase muscle mass, when performed in circuit or high-repetition formats, it significantly enhances endurance. This is especially important because muscular endurance is a core component of physical endurance. As your muscles adapt to handle longer periods of activity, so too can you handle prolonged intimate encounters without discomfort or fatigue.

Transforming fitness routines to focus on endurance doesn't just lead to physical benefits. It nourishes the mind as well. Exercise is a powerful tool for mental health, reducing symptoms of anxiety and depression—both of which can stifle libido. Exercise releases endorphins, the body's natural mood lifters, aiding a positive mindset. A brighter outlook can make you more receptive to intimacy, leading to more frequent and satisfying connections.

Moreover, the psychological boost from achieving fitness goals fosters confidence. Reaching new milestones builds self-esteem, encouraging a healthier body image and instilling the courage to embrace intimacy. Feeling good about oneself is a precursor to feeling good with someone else.

An often-overlooked aspect of endurance training is its ability to fortify resilience. When faced with difficult tasks, those with greater physical endurance often display improved problem-solving skills under stress. This resilience is invaluable when overcoming challenges in relationships or addressing personal health issues that impact libido.

Let's not disregard the social dimension of fitness. Joining a community for group exercises or sports can provide a sense of belonging, support and motivation. This helps not only in maintaining fitness but also in creating social connections that combat loneliness, subsequently enhancing one's overall well-being and readiness to engage in intimate relationships.

As you progress on your fitness journey, be mindful of measuring and celebrating improvements. Whether it's an increase in endurance, a faster pace, or simply feeling less fatigued throughout the day, recognising these achievements can be deeply motivating. Progress can reignite a sense of vitality, which can naturally extend to bolstering your libido.

In conclusion, the role of fitness in endurance is multifaceted with profound implications for sexual desire. Through enhancing cardiovascular health, hormonal balance, and mental resilience, endurance training provides a foundational boost to overall well-being. This, in turn, positively influences libido, creating a cycle of vitality and improved intimate experiences. By committing to an active lifestyle and embracing endurance-enhancing activities, you can unlock energy reserves capable of transforming not just your physical health, but the quality of your intimate relationships as well.

# Chapter 19:
# Tackling Age-Related
# Libido Challenges

Ageing doesn't mean waving goodbye to your libido; instead, it's an invitation to explore intimacy from a fresh perspective. As we age, our bodies and minds evolve, requiring us to adjust expectations and tailor solutions that resonate with our journeys. Embracing ageing positively begins with recognising that the wisdom and experience accumulated over the years can enrich your sexual well-being. Shift your focus from what's lost to what can be gained: a deeper emotional connection with your partner, patience, and understanding. With age, there comes an opportunity to redefine passion, integrating gentler approaches to intimacy that honour both physical and emotional changes. By doing so, you'll not only sustain but also enhance your relationship, turning potential challenges into pathways for growth. Being open to new experiences and maintaining an active dialogue with your partner can transform your intimate life, making it as fulfilling as ever. Adjusting expectations thoughtfully can lead to discovering new layers of satisfaction, proving that passion is indeed timeless.

## Embracing Ageing Positively

Ageing is an inevitable part of life, and it can bring with it a range of changes, both physical and emotional. However, embracing these changes positively can significantly impact one's overall well-being and relationship dynamics. As men grow older, the challenges related to libido can become more pronounced. Yet, by adopting a positive perspective on ageing, men and their partners can navigate these challenges with grace and compassion.

Understanding that ageing is a natural process is crucial. Accepting it doesn't mean relinquishing one's desire for intimacy, but rather reshaping how we perceive and engage with it. With age comes wisdom and a deeper understanding of oneself and one's partner, allowing for a more profound connection. Shifting focus from performance-based goals to shared experiences and mutual satisfaction can enhance relationships in unforeseen ways.

Society often presents ageing in a negative light, associating it with decline and loss. Yet, it's essential to challenge this narrative. In the context of sexual health and well-being, growing older can offer opportunities to explore new dimensions of intimacy and connection. This stage of life can be a time for discovery, as men and their partners learn to communicate their needs more openly and without judgement.

A vital aspect of ageing positively is fostering a supportive environment. Encouragement from a partner can be invaluable, and this support should be reciprocated. When couples face challenges tied to libido changes, having open and honest conversations can lead to greater understanding and intimacy. Together, they can redefine their relationship's sexual narrative, setting new benchmarks that honour their evolving desires and needs.

Additionally, ageing often brings about a shift in priorities, allowing individuals to focus on emotional connection over physical performance. The pressures to conform to youthful ideals diminish, making way for affection that is based on genuine connection and appreciation. This emotional warmth can lead to a more fulfilling and deeply satisfying partnership.

Embracing ageing also involves acknowledging and adapting to physical changes that occur with time. This could mean exploring different forms of sexual expression and finding joy in new experiences that were previously unexplored. Instead of viewing these adjustments as limitations, they can be seen as opportunities to learn and grow together, creating a more expansive view of intimacy and pleasure.

Moreover, staying physically active and maintaining a healthy lifestyle can enhance one's libido and overall well-being. Regular exercise, a balanced diet, and sufficient rest are integral components of a vibrant life, regardless of age. They contribute not only to physical health but also to mental and emotional resilience, which are essential when navigating the ups and downs of a long-term relationship.

Ageing positively also involves keeping an open mind and being willing to explore different avenues for enhancing pleasure and intimacy. This openness can sometimes lead to the discovery of new techniques or perspectives that are particularly suited to one's changing body and desires. By remaining curious and adaptable, men and their partners can continue to cultivate a dynamic and satisfying intimate connection.

Crucially, embracing ageing positively is about self-compassion. It's about recognising that changes in libido are a normal part of getting older and not a reflection of one's worth or desirability. Letting go of self-criticism and instead focusing on self-acceptance and love can have profound effects on a person's confidence and outlook.

Partners play a crucial role in this aspect as well. By nurturing an environment of mutual support and understanding, couples can foster a relationship that is both resilient and rewarding. Acts of kindness, thoughtfulness, and tenderness should form the foundation of their interactions, reinforcing the bond that transcends physical changes.

Ultimately, embracing ageing positively requires a shift in perspective—away from a focus on limitations and towards an attitude of appreciation and growth. By opening themselves up to the possibilities that each stage of life brings, individuals and couples can experience a renewed sense of joy and fulfilment, extending beyond any challenges they may face. This positive mindset can transform not only how they view themselves but also how they relate to their partners, paving the way for a vibrant and enduring connection.

## Adjusting Expectations

As men age, certain changes are inevitable, and one of the most significant adjustments often involves recalibrating expectations around sexual desire and performance. It's perfectly natural to experience shifts in libido as the years progress, but these changes shouldn't be seen as diminishing one's value or capability. Instead, they can be approached as an opportunity to redefine what intimacy and satisfaction mean in this new stage of life.

Understanding that libido isn't a static attribute is crucial. Just as our bodies change over time, so too can our sexual appetites. This doesn't mean resignation to a lacklustre intimate life, but rather an invitation to explore new dimensions of connection and pleasure. Accepting these shifts allows couples to embark on a journey of learning and adaptation, which can ultimately deepen their bond and enhance their relationship.

Many who struggle with a decline in libido fear that they are somehow less, or that their relationships are destined to suffer as a result. However, these feelings often stem from societal pressures that promote a narrow view of sexuality. It's essential to challenge these outdated norms and recognise that fulfillment and satisfaction can come from a variety of experiences beyond just physical intimacy. A partnership thriving on mutual understanding and shared growth can be incredibly rewarding, regardless of the frequency or intensity of sexual encounters.

One crucial aspect of adjusting expectations is acknowledging that age-related changes in libido are a common experience. Numerous factors contribute to this, including hormonal shifts, changes in health, and alterations in relationship dynamics. By recognising these elements, individuals can begin to see their sexual journey as a complex interplay of forces rather than a straightforward decline. This perspective fosters a more compassionate self-view and realistic expectations, paving the way for healthier relationships.

Moreover, embracing age gracefully involves appreciating the wisdom that comes with experience. Many find that with age comes a broader understanding of intimacy and the many forms it can take. This shift can lead to discovering new ways to express desire, love, and connection that may not have been considered in younger years. For instance, focusing on emotional intimacy, communication, and shared activities can bring partners closer together and reignite passion in unexpected ways.

It's also essential to consider the role of external pressures and how they may shape one's expectations and perceptions. Media portrayal of sexuality often glosses over the reality of ageing, creating an unrealistic standard for many. By critically evaluating these influences and separating them from personal beliefs, individuals can develop a healthier, more authentic view of their sexual selves. This process involves not just individual reflection but also honest conversations with partners to align on shared expectations and desires.

At times, adjusting expectations may include seeking professional guidance. Consulting with healthcare providers or therapists can provide valuable insights into the physical and psychological aspects of libido decline. These professionals can offer strategies tailored to one's specific needs, helping to address any underlying issues and facilitate productive discussions with partners. Such interventions not only help manage expectations but also empower individuals and couples to take control of their sexual health and well-being.

It's also important to note that adjusting expectations doesn't entail lowering them to a point where one gives up on intimacy altogether. Rather, it's about redefining what satisfaction looks like and finding joy in different moments and experiences. This might include more frequent displays of affection, exploring new forms of intimacy, or simply enjoying the comfort of companionship. Each couple has the opportunity to define what works best for them, free from the constraints of conventional expectations.

For those who find themselves struggling with these adjustments, there is immense power in community and shared experiences. Connecting with others who are facing similar challenges can provide not only support but also a wealth of practical advice and personal insights. Many men find solace and inspiration in knowing they are not alone in this journey, and sharing their stories can spark new approaches and ideas.

Acknowledging and adjusting expectations around age-related libido changes is a process that requires patience and openness. It's not always easy to confront one's shifting desires or to discuss these changes with a partner, but doing so can lead to a more enriched, meaningful connection. By taking this step with an open mind and heart, individuals can navigate this transition with grace and enthusiasm, ultimately fostering a deeper appreciation for the richness of later-life intimacy.

## Tailoring Solutions for Older Adults

As we delve into the intricacies of libido, it's imperative to acknowledge the unique challenges that older adults face. Ageing brings a host of physical and emotional changes, many of which can impact sexual desire. However, it's crucial to understand that a decline in libido is not an inevitable part of ageing. With the right approach, older adults can continue to experience fulfilling, passionate relationships.

One of the first steps in tailoring solutions for older adults is recognising the changing landscape of their bodies. As the body ages, hormonal shifts, particularly a decrease in testosterone for men, can significantly affect libido. Hormonal therapy might be a viable option for some, but it's essential to consult with a healthcare provider to understand the benefits and risks involved. It's not just about replacing what's lost but understanding the body's new rhythm and finding ways to harmonise with it.

Besides hormonal changes, physical health conditions like cardiovascular issues, diabetes, and arthritis are more prevalent among older adults and can affect sexual function. Addressing these conditions with a healthcare provider can not only improve overall health but also enhance sexual well-being. Effective management of such conditions often leads to improvements in energy levels, self-esteem, and libido. Exercise, alongside appropriate medical treatments, remains a cornerstone of maintaining sexual health in older age.

While physical health is vital, we mustn't overlook the power of the mind. Older adults may face psychological hurdles such as anxiety, depression, or body image issues, which can dampen sexual desire. Open dialogue with partners and professionals can alleviate these concerns. The act of sharing one's fears and insecurities can lead to deeper emotional bonds and reduced anxiety. In this stage of life, relationships built on honesty and understanding often reap significant benefits.

Communication plays a pivotal role in addressing age-related libido challenges. Discussing this aspect of life openly with one's partner encourages a supportive environment where both parties feel valued and heard. It's important to redefine intimacy beyond just the physical act; emotional and intellectual connections can foster a satisfying sexual relationship. Exploring ways to express love and affection outside the bedroom can enrich the couple's connection, paving the way for a more relaxed and enjoyable sexual experience when the time comes.

Exploration of new methods and tools is another key strategy. As we age, what might have worked in the past may no longer be effective or satisfying. This period of life can be an opportunity to explore new avenues of pleasure, be it through sensual massages, different positions, or even sex toys, if desired. Embracing novelty without fear of judgment or failure often leads to surprising discoveries and rekindles the excitement.

Educational resources also provide a wealth of information tailored specifically for older adults. Books, workshops, and seminars aimed at mature audiences can offer insights into sexual health and innovations. Gaining knowledge about what's happening to your body and how best to care for it empowers older adults to make informed decisions about their sexual health.

Moreover, the role of diet and nutrition cannot be underestimated. A well-balanced diet that includes foods known to enhance libido, like nuts, seeds, and dark chocolate, can make a difference. Ensuring sufficient intake of vitamins and minerals, especially those that boost energy and mood, supports sexual health. For many older adults, simple changes in diet can lead to profound improvements in health and libido.

Maintaining a healthy lifestyle is about more than just diet. Adequate sleep, staying hydrated, reducing alcohol consumption, and avoiding smoking are critical factors. Together, they create a holistic approach that supports sexual health. These changes complement medical and psychological interventions, providing a well-rounded approach to enhancing libido.

For some, engaging in therapeutic practices might be beneficial. Counselling or therapy, either individually or as a couple, can offer strategies for managing specific sexual concerns or relational dynamics. These sessions provide a safe space to explore desires, conflicts, and expectations, ultimately resulting in stronger intimacy and connection.

Ultimately, the journey of maintaining and enhancing sexual desire in older age is as unique as the individuals embarking on it. It requires a blend of strategy, communication, exploration, and self-care. By embracing the changes that come with age positively and adjusting expectations accordingly, older adults can continue to enjoy love, passion, and companionship.

The key is understanding that time brings growth and wisdom, allowing a deepening appreciation for intimacy in all its forms. This chapter of life offers the chance to redefine what sexual fulfillment means and to cultivate relationships that continue to thrive with tenderness and love. With an open mind and a willing heart, the possibilities for passionate and meaningful connections remain as vibrant as ever, regardless of age.

# Chapter 20:
# Evaluating and Adjusting
# Belief Systems

In this chapter, we're delving into the profound impact that belief systems have on libido and intimacy. Often, the mind's unyielding grip on entrenched beliefs can unknowingly curb sexual desire and stall relationship growth. Identifying limiting beliefs is the first crucial step on the journey towards a richer, more fulfilling intimate life. Envision these beliefs as hidden scripts that can dictate one's responses and feelings towards intimacy. By applying a growth mindset, which is the willingness to embrace change and learn from experiences, you can gradually dismantle these barriers and cultivate a landscape ripe for personal and relational transformation. It's about developing positive attitudes that not only encourage a healthy self-image but also bolster confidence and openness, essential for restoring desire and connection. So, break free from old narratives, and seek perspectives that inspire resilience and positivity—this adjustment can be a cornerstone in reigniting passion in your relationship.

## Identifying Limiting Beliefs

Beliefs shape our reality in profound ways. They carve out the path we walk, influencing every aspect of our lives, from mundane daily decisions to significant life choices. Yet, when these beliefs become limiting, they can cage us in, stalling progress and stifling potential. For men experiencing a decline in sexual desire, these invisible barriers may lurk in the shadows, unnamed and unchallenged. Understanding and identifying these limiting beliefs is crucial for reigniting passion and nurturing a healthier, more fulfilling intimate relationship.

Limiting beliefs often develop subtly, blending into one's psyche as truths. They manifest in the silent dialogues we have with ourselves, shaping perceptions of our sexual capabilities, desirability, and relational value. Common examples include beliefs like "I'm too old for intimacy" or "My partner just isn't interested in me anymore". Such thoughts can spiral into self-fulfilling prophecies, undermining confidence and eroding the bedrock of a satisfying sexual life.

A powerful starting point in tackling these beliefs is self-awareness. Self-reflection allows individuals to pierce the veil of false narratives that cloud judgment and decision-making. Reflecting on where these beliefs started can be enlightening. Often, they emerge from past experiences, societal norms, or inaccurate portrayals of masculinity and sexuality. For some, a voice of criticism or doubt from past relationships may loom large, casting a long shadow over present interactions.

External influences also play a significant role. Cultural and societal norms can impose rigid expectations about sexual vitality and performance. The media often presents an idealised vision of sexual prowess, one that is persistent, unwavering, and frequently unattainable. For many men, this can lead to feelings of inadequacy or pressure, breeding beliefs that they cannot measure up. Understanding the impact of these influences helps to untether from unrealistic standards, opening the door to developing a more personal and authentic understanding of sexuality.

Challenging these beliefs requires courage and honesty. It's about questioning the narratives that have been accepted without scrutiny. Ask yourself, "Is this belief serving me?", "Where did it come from?", and critically, "Is it truly accurate?" Such introspection can lead to revelations that liberate and empower. While this journey might feel confronting, it's equally invigorating, allowing space for growth and transformation.

The next step is replacing those constraining beliefs with more supportive, empowering ones. This isn't just about positive thinking but about embracing a mindset that reflects flexibility, realism, and optimism. Consider adopting beliefs like "I'm capable of growth and improvement" or "Intimacy is a shared journey, not a performance". Such shifts in perspective can profoundly impact how one perceives sexual interactions and relationships.

Breaking free from limiting beliefs doesn't happen overnight. It's a process that involves not only recognising and addressing the beliefs themselves but also frequent reinforcement of new, healthier narratives. Developing strategies such as journaling, discussing with a trusted partner or friend, and practising mindfulness can aid in this ongoing transformation. Each tool offers a way to gain clarity, express emotions, and reaffirm commitment to a new path.

Partners can play a pivotal role in this process too. Open and honest dialogue forms the backbone of mutual support and understanding. By sharing their experiences and perspectives, partners can dispel fears and anxieties that feed limiting beliefs. This mutual sharing not only strengthens the bond but also builds a safe space for vulnerability and acceptance, enabling both partners to explore and express their desires without fear of judgment or rejection.

Moreover, professional guidance from therapists or counsellors can offer invaluable insight and strategies. These professionals provide an objective lens, helping individuals to see past the fog of entrenched beliefs and nurture a renewed sense of sexual confidence and connection. They offer customised approaches that resonate with the individual's unique life experience, encouraging small, sustainable steps toward change.

This path of identifying and overcoming limiting beliefs is ultimately about liberation. It's about reclaiming sexual desire and intimacy as a vibrant, life-affirming part of oneself, free from the shackles of unrealistic expectations or past disappointments. By addressing these beliefs with intention and sincerity, individuals can pave the way toward a more authentic, satisfying, and enriching intimate life.

In this journey, remember that growth stems from motion, from the willingness to confront discomfort and to face the unknown with an open heart. Embrace this exploration not just as a means to restore sexual desire but as an opportunity to deepen your understanding of yourself and your relationship. Let the collapsing of these barriers be a catalyst for a richer, more diverse expression of intimacy that honours where you've been and where you aspire to go.

## Embracing Growth Mindset

In our journey to evaluating and adjusting belief systems, embracing a growth mindset stands as a pivotal element. The concept, rooted in the belief that abilities and intelligence can be developed with time and effort, offers a refreshing perspective on tackling libido challenges. A growth mindset encourages us to view obstacles not as impenetrable walls, but as opportunities for learning and improvement. When it comes to declining sexual desire, this mindset shifts the focus from frustration and resignation to curiosity and perseverance.

Adopting a growth mindset requires a change in our internal dialogue. Consider the way we talk to ourselves when faced with a challenge in intimacy. Many of us might default to thoughts filled with self-doubt or blame. This negative self-talk acts as a significant barrier to progress. By transforming these thoughts into constructive ones, such as "What can I learn from this?" or "How can I improve?" we start to open doors to new possibilities. This shift in thinking fosters resilience, allowing us to approach issues in our relationship with greater patience and creativity.

It's important to remember that a growth mindset isn't a quick fix, nor is it a denial of the difficulties faced. It's about accepting that while the path might be rough, we have the capacity to navigate it successfully. When dealing with libido loss, this perspective can mitigate some of the helplessness and anxiety often associated with the issue. It shifts focus from what we perceive as innate shortcomings to a realm of strategy and empowerment. Sexual desire becomes something dynamic, subject to enhancement and growth, rather than a fixed trait we feel victimised by.

Couples can foster a shared growth mindset to strengthen their relationship. Open communication is key here. Conversations that involve mutual vulnerability and a willingness to learn from each other can significantly enhance emotional intimacy. Couples should discuss their challenges without judgement and work together to identify strengths as well as areas for growth. A relationship is a living entity, and as such, it's meant to evolve. Understanding this helps partners support each other through the natural ebbs and flows of desire.

Emphasising growth becomes particularly empowering in the bedroom. Instead of focusing on performance and outcome, engaging in exploration and play can unlock new dimensions of intimacy. Trying new approaches, experimenting with different methods of connection, and recognising that setbacks are merely steps in the learning process cultivates a richer sexual experience. With a growth mindset, each encounter becomes a chance to deepen understanding and improve connection, turning challenges into shared journeys.

Real-world examples provide evidence of how transformative a growth mindset can be. Consider a couple who've been struggling with decreased passion. By shifting their focus from "fixing a problem" to "exploring new possibilities," they begin approaching their intimate life as a shared adventure. This change results in reduced pressure, allowing them to rediscover each other in unexpected ways. Their focus on growth over perfection brings a sense of playfulness and anticipation back into their lives.

Developing a growth mindset also requires personal accountability, where each partner takes responsibility for their own development. This independence enables partners to contribute equally to the relationship's growth. Engaging in self-reflection and setting personal goals can drive change from within. Perhaps it's committing to learning more about personal sexual satisfaction, or setting realistic goals to improve oneself in the context of intimacy.

Furthermore, a growth mindset invites a broader view of self-improvement, encompassing emotional, intellectual, and physical dimensions. It promotes a holistic approach, encouraging practices that don't solely focus on immediate desire but enhance overall wellness. By taking care of one's mental health, physical health, and spiritual balance, a person creates a fertile ground for desire to flourish. Each of these aspects contributes to personal growth that naturally enhances sexual experiences.

Now, you may wonder, how do you nurture this mindset effectively? Begin with mindfulness. Practicing mindfulness fosters an awareness of present experiences without judgment. It helps individuals stay connected with their thoughts and emotions, allowing them to alter negative patterns and embrace positive growth-focused thinking. Whether through meditation, journaling, or reflective conversations, mindfulness acts as a catalyst for sustaining a growth mindset.

Also essential is the power of patience. Embracing a growth mindset doesn't mean rushing change; it's about steady progression. Encourage patience both within yourself and your partner. Allow space for experimentation and the inevitable learning that comes through trial and error. Recognise that not every attempt will yield immediate results, but each experience provides valuable insights that contribute to long-term growth.

Sometimes, professional guidance can further reinforce this mindset. Therapy or counselling can provide a supportive environment where individuals and couples learn to identify and overcome limiting beliefs. Therapists can serve as facilitators who help partners adopt a perspective focused on growth, challenge, and resilience. This support often extends into practical advice and strategies tailored to individual needs and contexts.

As you progress in this journey, it's crucial to celebrate small victories. Acknowledging progress, no matter how minor, reinforces motivation and confidence. Whether it's newfound openness in communication, a deeper emotional connection, or an innovative step in intimacy, recognising these achievements is vital. They serve as reminders of one's capability to grow and make meaningful changes, reinforcing the mindset's positive impact.

Ultimately, embracing a growth mindset aligns perfectly with the overall goal of addressing libido loss: not just to restore desire but to transform relationships into more fulfilling and dynamic experiences. By focusing on potential rather than limitation, we empower ourselves and our partners to adapt, learn, and thrive together. In making this shift, we encourage a journey defined by shared exploration, mutual learning, and enriched emotional bonds.

## Developing Positive Attitudes

Attitudes shape our perception of the world and deeply influence our interactions and decisions. When it comes to sexual desire and relationships, cultivating a positive attitude is crucial. It's about shifting perspectives, broadening horizons, and embracing the possibility of change. Positive attitudes can transform the landscape of an otherwise dwindling relationship by injecting hope and enthusiasm, providing the groundwork for rejuvenating intimacy.

Adopting a positive mindset doesn't mean ignoring the difficulties encountered. Rather, it involves recognising challenges for what they are and actively seeking ways to overcome them. Many men and their partners facing a decline in sexual desire often find themselves mired in a cycle of negativity, which only exacerbates the issue. Breaking this cycle requires acknowledging the problem without judgment and deliberately choosing to approach solutions with optimism.

A crucial step is reframing the narrative surrounding libido loss. Instead of viewing it as a sign of failure or inadequacy, consider it an opportunity for growth and deeper connection. By shifting the focus from what's wrong to what's possible, couples can open themselves up to new experiences and solutions previously overlooked. Changing the way we think about issues can often be just as transformative as the actions we take to address them.

In relationships, the encouragement and support of a partner play a significant role in developing positive attitudes. It's about building each other up and fostering an environment where both parties feel empowered to express their desires, fears, and aspirations without fear of ridicule. The foundation of this positive environment is effective communication, which involves more than just words. It's about empathy, patience, and the willingness to truly listen.

Developing a positive attitude also involves being gentle with oneself. Self-criticism can be debilitating, and when it comes to issues like libido loss, it's easy to fall into the trap of self-blame. Learning to practice self-compassion, recognising that everyone experiences ups and downs, and that seeking help is a strength rather than a weakness is essential. Embracing personal imperfections and viewing them as part of the human experience can dramatically shift one's mindset.

Beyond self-compassion, setting realistic expectations can greatly influence attitude. Understanding that changes may take time and that not every attempt will result in immediate success can prevent unnecessary frustration. The key is persistence and the courage to keep moving forward even when progress feels slow. Celebrating small victories along the way, such as open conversations or newly discovered shared interests, can reinforce a positive outlook.

Cultivating gratitude is another powerful tool in developing positive attitudes. Regularly acknowledging and appreciating the strengths in oneself and one's partner can foster a sense of contentment and joy. This doesn't mean ignoring issues that need addressing but rather balancing constructive efforts with recognition of what's going well. Gratitude can serve as a reminder of the love and connection that brought the relationship together initially, which often gets forgotten over time.

Physical activity and mindfulness practices can also support the development of a positive mindset. Activities that connect the mind and body, such as yoga or tai chi, encourage present-moment awareness and can reduce stress and anxiety, which often hinder positive attitudes. When the mind is calm and present, it's easier to approach challenges with clarity and optimism.

As individuals work on fostering positive attitudes, it's essential to remember that this is an ongoing process. Attitudes can fluctuate, and maintaining positivity requires regular nurturing. Engaging with material that inspires, whether books, podcasts, or conversations with friends, can keep one motivated. Surrounding oneself with people who embody positivity is equally important, as their enthusiasm can be contagious.

Finally, embracing the concept of a growth mindset underpins the development of positive attitudes. This involves recognising that abilities and circumstances can be improved with effort over time.

Viewing setbacks as opportunities for learning rather than as insurmountable obstacles encourages resilience. With a growth mindset, the journey of addressing libido loss becomes a path of personal and relational development, strengthening bonds and deepening intimacy.

In conclusion, developing positive attitudes requires conscious effort and a willingness to adapt and evolve. It's about seeing challenges as chances to grow, engaging in open and supportive communication, fostering gratitude, and practicing self-compassion. By adjusting belief systems and embracing positivity, individuals and couples can revive their connection, rekindle their passion, and move towards a deeper, more fulfilling relationship.

# Chapter 21:
## Dealing with Performance Anxiety

Performance anxiety can act like an invisible barrier, casting a shadow over intimate moments and turning anticipation into apprehension. It's not just a physical challenge; it's an emotional echo that resonates through the mind, body, and even extends to the dynamics of a relationship. Often rooted in the pressures to meet perceived expectations, this anxiety can be as much about the fear of not measuring up as it is about the act itself. But there's hope and a way forward. Embracing strategies that focus on open communication, self-compassion, and realistic goal-setting can help dismantle these pressures, turning vulnerability into a shared opportunity for growth. Professionals in the field suggest tailored approaches, combining mindfulness and therapeutic guidance, as effective tools to recalibrate perspectives and rebuild confidence. By demystifying and addressing performance anxiety, there's a chance not only to alleviate its impact but to rediscover joy in connection—an endeavour that enriches both personal and shared experiences. Remember, it's about progress, not perfection, and each step towards overcoming this hurdle is a testament to resilience and commitment to a fulfilling intimate life.

## Understanding Its Origins

Performance anxiety, particularly in intimate situations, can be a labyrinth of emotions and psychological hurdles. Pinpointing its roots requires a deep dive into its various contributing factors, which often intertwine. For many men, this anxiety creeps in during the most inopportune moments, casting a shadow over times meant for connection and joy. And what's often misunderstood is that the origin of performance anxiety is rarely a single incident or cause. It's often a confluence of experiences, perceptions, and even societal pressures that manifest during intimate moments.

Many men carry the weight of societal expectations about virility and sexual prowess. From a young age, boys absorb stereotypes that equate masculinity with unyielding strength and performance. While these images might seem like harmless cultural norms, they embed deeply held beliefs that to be a man means to be always 'ready' and effective in intimate settings. These beliefs can pile up silently over the years, unnoticed until an unexpected moment of vulnerability triggers anxiety.

Past experiences can also lay the groundwork for performance anxiety. A previously awkward or disappointing intimate encounter can linger in a man's psyche, casting doubt over future possibilities. This self-doubt perpetuates a vicious cycle, where the fear of repeating past mistakes creates even more anxiety, leading to decreased performance and satisfaction. It's a feedback loop that can be hard to break without understanding its origins.

Beyond personal history, broader psychological contributors also have a role to play. Stress, depression, and other mental health issues, as explored in earlier chapters, significantly impact a person's sexual performance and desire. When the mind is under constant pressure, it prioritises survival and coping mechanisms over pleasure and relaxation. This diversion can strip away the vital aspects of spontaneity and connection in intimate situations, replacing them with dread and pressure.

Physical health shouldn't be overlooked when considering the origins of performance anxiety. Conditions like diabetes, heart disease, or hormonal imbalances can affect sexual function, creating anxiety around performance. The fear of a physiological limitation transforming into a real-time challenge undermines confidence. Yet often, this is exacerbated by a lack of understanding that the mind and body are intricately interconnected.

The relationship dynamics and the environment in which intimacy occurs are equally crucial. A history of unresolved conflicts, poor communication, or lack of emotional support from a partner can contribute to feelings of inadequacy and fear. Partners play a pivotal role in either soothing these fears or, unfortunately, amplifying them. Understanding this shared aspect is essential to addressing the roots of performance anxiety.

Moreover, cultural and media influences cannot be ignored. The portrayal of sexual encounters in media often sets unrealistic standards and expectations, leading men to question their adequacy and prowess. This bombardment can lead to comparing real-life experiences with fantasy, fostering the seeds of doubt and anxiety. Recognising that these portrayals are exaggerations rather than benchmarks is vital in reclaiming one's sexual confidence.

Understanding the origins of performance anxiety requires delving into self-perception and self-worth. Men's identities are often closely tied to their perceived sexual capabilities. When performance anxiety strikes, it challenges these core beliefs, shaking confidence to its foundation. This makes it imperative to separate one's self-worth from performance metrics, focusing on factors like kindness, partnership, and genuine connection instead.

Lastly, familial and cultural upbringing can leave lasting imprints on how men perceive their roles in relationships. Specific cultures place a high emphasis on male dominance and sexual conquer, which can be stifling for those who fail to measure up to these arbitrary standards. Overcoming these ingrained beliefs involves a journey of introspection and sometimes professional guidance to reshape these narratives into healthier, more achievable perspectives.

In summing up, understanding the origins of performance anxiety is multifaceted, rooted in personal history, psychological factors, physical health, cultural influences, and self-perceptions. The process of unraveling these threads requires patience and honest self-reflection, as well as an openness to seek support when needed. By addressing these complex origins, men can begin to dismantle the walls that performance anxiety builds and move towards more fulfilling and intimate connections.

## Strategies to Alleviate Pressures

Performance anxiety can feel like a shadow casting itself over intimate moments, making them less about connection and more about self-doubt. However, understanding this common barrier is the first step in alleviating its pressures. It's crucial to appreciate that such anxiety often stems from a fear of judgement or failure. This fear can arise from past experiences, media portrayals, or personal insecurities, leading to a spiralling effect that impacts libido and sexual performance.

One effective strategy to relieve this pressure is reframing the narrative surrounding sexual encounters. Rather than focusing on achieving a specific outcome, shift the emphasis to the process and the enjoyment of the moment. Viewing intimacy as an opportunity to connect rather than perform can reduce anxiety and promote a more relaxed and authentic experience. This mindset shift often requires patience and self-compassion, along with open communication with one's partner.

Another approach involves integrating relaxation techniques into one's routine. Breathing exercises, meditation, and mindfulness practices can help in reducing overall stress levels. These techniques engage the parasympathetic nervous system, nurturing a sense of calm and reducing the body's fight-or-flight response that performance anxiety often triggers. Practising these regularly can make the bedroom feel like a haven rather than a stage.

Visualisation can also be an empowering tool. Imagining a positive and fulfilling intimate encounter not only boosts confidence but also helps in setting a positive expectation. Doing this can gradually replace anxiety-laden thoughts with ones filled with excitement and anticipation. Over time, this can create a new mental map that favours positive experiences, reducing the pressure to perform and increasing the enjoyment of the experience.

Furthermore, setting realistic expectations is crucial. Unrealistic ideals about performance, driven by societal norms or media portrayals, can exacerbate anxiety. Recognising that every individual and every couple is different helps in setting expectations that honour personal experiences and dynamics. Discussing these expectations with a partner ensures mutual understanding, thereby reducing both individual and shared pressure.

Building confidence outside the bedroom can significantly impact performance anxiety. Engaging in activities that bolster self-esteem and cultivate a positive self-image can work wonders. Whether it's through exercise, developing new skills, or nurturing hobbies, feeling good about oneself translates into reduced anxieties in intimate settings. Confidence can be contagious, creating a more relaxed and enthusiastic approach to intimacy.

Learning to focus on the present rather than worrying about performance can dramatically alleviate anxiety. Training oneself to engage fully with current sensations and emotions helps in quietening the critical inner dialogue that often accompanies performance anxiety. Being present in the moment allows natural chemistry and connection to unfold, offering richer and more fulfilling experiences.

Addressing underlying emotional issues and insecurities is also fundamental. Personal fears or previous traumas can manifest as anxiety in intimate moments. Therapy or counselling provides a safe environment to explore these issues, offering professional insights and guidance. This can be a pivotal step towards healing and finding a path beyond performance anxiety.

Partners play a vital role in alleviating performance anxiety pressures. Creating a supportive and understanding environment encourages open dialogues about worries and fears. This foundation of trust allows for shared solutions and offers reassurance that performance isn't the sole focus of an encounter. A partner's empathy can be a powerful balm, reaffirming that love and connection transcend performance metrics.

Lastly, reducing performance anxiety involves embracing vulnerability. It is through vulnerability that deeper connections are formed. By allowing oneself to be seen and accepted for who they truly are, without the fear of judgement or ridicule, intimate experiences can become more authentic and rewarding. This openness fosters intimacy in its truest form, shifting focus from performing to connecting.

In conclusion, addressing performance anxiety requires a multifaceted approach that involves self-reflection, support, and practical strategies. By shifting perspectives, engaging in relaxation practices, setting realistic expectations, and fostering open communication, one can transform anxiety into an opportunity for growth and deeper connection. Embracing vulnerability alongside a supportive partner paves the way for richer and more meaningful intimate experiences, ultimately alleviating the pressures that once loomed large. These steps, both personal and shared, can ease the distress of performance anxiety, paving the way for a more fulfilling and liberated intimate life.

## Professional Insights and Help

Performance anxiety, particularly in intimate settings, can feel like a daunting mountain to climb. For many men, it saps the joy out of relationships, affecting both partners emotionally and physically. Professional insights and targeted help can offer a beacon of hope, transforming seemingly insurmountable challenges into manageable landscapes. Let's delve into how seeking professional assistance can be a game-changer in addressing performance anxiety, offering both practical solutions and profound insights.

Firstly, understanding the origins of performance anxiety is crucial. It's often tied to deeper psychological roots, such as fear of inadequacy, past experiences, or societal pressures that dictate what it means to be 'manly'. Professional therapists and counsellors can provide a safe, unbiased space to explore these underlying issues. By unpacking complex emotions and experiences with a non-judgmental professional, men can begin to dismantle the mental barriers contributing to their anxiety. This process not only aids in overcoming anxiety but also fosters greater self-awareness, which is integral to personal growth.

Therapists often work collaboratively with clients to identify specific triggers of performance anxiety. Through techniques such as cognitive behavioural therapy (CBT), they can help reframe negative thought patterns into positive ones. CBT is particularly effective in helping individuals challenge and change unhelpful cognitions about performance, promoting healthier attitudes and coping mechanisms. This shift in mindset can significantly diminish anxiety, leading to improved performance and enhanced satisfaction in intimate encounters.

Besides traditional psychotherapy, some men might benefit from exploring alternative therapeutic options. Hypnotherapy, for instance, uses guided relaxation and focused attention to help individuals tap into their subconscious, potentially uncovering and resolving deep-seated anxiety causes. While the effectiveness of such treatments can vary from person to person, they offer additional avenues for exploration, especially for those who might not respond to conventional methods.

Moreover, professionals can offer valuable insights into the physiological aspects of performance anxiety. Stress-induced physiological responses, such as an increased heart rate and adrenaline surge, can exacerbate feelings of anxiety. Understanding these physical responses can empower men to adopt techniques to manage them more effectively. Breathing exercises or mindfulness practices, for example, can help ground individuals in the present moment, reducing anxiety and improving focus during intimate moments.

Couples' therapy is another critical avenue to explore. Performance anxiety doesn't just affect the individual experiencing it; it impacts the relationship as a whole. Partners may inadvertently add pressure, or themselves struggle with feelings of inadequacy or rejection. Couples' therapy provides a forum for open dialogue, fostering understanding and empathy. Therapists can guide conversations in a way that promotes mutual support and collective problem-solving, thus strengthening the emotional bond between partners.

Furthermore, clear, empathetic communication facilitated by a professional can help partners better articulate their needs and anxieties. Encouraging open and honest discussions reduces misunderstandings and enhances emotional intimacy. When partners understand the role of anxiety and work together towards solutions, performance anxiety can become an opportunity to grow closer, rather than a wedge driven between them.

In some cases, exploring medical interventions might be necessary. Professionals, such as urologists or endocrinologists, can assess if there's a physiological factor exacerbating performance anxiety. Evaluating testosterone levels, checking for underlying medical conditions, or adjusting current medications could also play a part. Addressing these health aspects under professional guidance can ease anxiety and improve overall wellness.

Integrating these professional insights with lifestyle changes can amplify positive outcomes. Regular follow-ups and check-ins with the professional can ensure ongoing support and accountability, reinforcing progress and providing a framework for tackling future challenges. This ongoing relationship with a professional can offer reassurance and boost confidence as progress is made.

At its core, the journey of overcoming performance anxiety with professional help is about building resilience. It's about learning to respond to stressors with calmness and clarity, cultivating a sense of control and empowerment. Professionals don't just provide quick fixes; they offer the tools to navigate anxiety effectively and sustainably, enhancing the quality of intimate relationships.

Men experiencing performance anxiety should remember that seeking help is not a sign of weakness, but rather a bold step towards regaining control of their lives and relationships. Through professional guidance, they can transform anxiety into an opportunity— reinforcing their capabilities, enriching their relationships, and creating a fulfilling, intimate life.

# Chapter 22:
## Engaging in Open Dialogue

Engaging in open dialogue is crucial for men experiencing a decline in sexual desire and their partners yearning for restored intimacy. Initiating candid conversations fosters a safe space where concerns can be expressed without judgment, ensuring both partners feel heard and valued. Breaking down barriers of shame and stigma requires vulnerability, yet it paves the way for deeper understanding and connection. It's about harnessing the courage to voice fears and desires while honing the art of attentive listening and constructive feedback. Through open dialogue, couples can dismantle misconceptions and build a foundation of trust that supports their journey towards renewed passion and a thriving relationship. Remember, the key lies in patience and empathy, as these conversations unfold naturally, strengthening the bonds that tie partners closer together.

### Creating a Safe Space for Communication

Building a safe environment for open dialogue can transform your relationship in ways you might not have thought possible. It's essential to understand that the root of many issues related to decreased sexual desire lies not only in physical or psychological factors but often in the way couples communicate—or fail to do so. Creating that secure and nurturing space for conversation helps to forge deeper connections, eliminate misunderstandings, and empower both partners to share their thoughts and feelings freely without judgement or fear. This section will guide you through the foundational steps required to foster such a transformative communicative space.

The cornerstone of any successful relationship, especially when dealing with sensitive issues like libido loss, is trust. Yet, trust is not merely granted; it must be continuously earned and nurtured through conscious and consistent efforts. When couples commit to communicating openly and honestly, they pave the way for a relationship that can endure challenges and grow stronger. Establishing trust begins with being vulnerable and showing your partner that it's okay to express fears, desires, and worries. This can be fortified through small acts of honesty and understanding that gradually build a robust support system where both partners feel secure.

Imagine a space where you can lay bare your innermost thoughts without the fear of misunderstanding. Achieving this involves setting the right tone before any discussion. Approach the conversation with respect and empathy, acknowledging that your partner's feelings are valid and important. Engage in active listening, reading both verbal and non-verbal cues, and avoid interrupting or dismissing their experiences. This practice doesn't only apply to discussions about libido but should be a fundamental principle in all interactions. By cultivating empathy and validation, you contribute to an environment where honest dialogue can flourish.

Respect is instrumental in creating a safe communicative space. Each person's perspective is shaped by their unique experiences, and acknowledging this diversity is critical. This involves accepting differences and negotiating those differences with a sense of fairness and understanding. When disagreements arise—an inevitable part of any healthy relationship—it's crucial to manage them constructively. Employ techniques such as negotiation and compromise, which can turn potential conflicts into opportunities for growth and deeper understanding of each other's needs and boundaries.

Regular conversations can be an avenue to continually reinforce the safety of this space. Set aside dedicated time for communication—perhaps a weekly or monthly check-in—to address concerns or changes in feelings or situations. It's essential to avoid having these important conversations in moments of heightened emotion or stress. Instead, choose calm, uninterrupted periods where both partners can focus on the dialogue. Regular dialogues can prevent miscommunications from snowballing into larger issues and help maintain a steady pulse on the relationship's health.

Physical space also plays a crucial role in communication. Choose environments that promote comfort and intimacy, free from distractions and stressors. Whether it's a quiet corner of your home or a favourite spot outside, the setting should invite openness and relaxation. A soothing atmosphere encourages openness, making it easier to tackle issues that you might otherwise find difficult to discuss.

Language matters, too—both the words and the tone you use can either open or shut doors to effective communication. Use language that invites discussion rather than criticism, focusing on "I" statements rather than "you" accusations. This approach minimises defensiveness and keeps the conversation rooted in personal experiences and feelings rather than blame. An example could be expressing, "I feel worried about our current level of intimacy," rather than, "You never seem interested anymore."

Building a new paradigm of communication often involves breaking down pre-existing barriers. Societal norms, upbringing, and past relationship experiences can all contribute to how you communicate. Recognising these barriers within yourself is as crucial as recognising them in your partner. Self-awareness promotes a deeper understanding of why certain topics feel difficult or why specific discussions lead to heightened emotional responses. By identifying and discussing these barriers, couples can dismantle them together, paving the way for more genuine interactions.

Finding solutions together is a key part of maintaining a safe communicative environment. When discussing issues like decreased libido, focus on resolving them together rather than placing the burden on one person. Brainstorming possible solutions or compromises reinforces the team aspect of your relationship and can catalyse collective problem-solving and creativity. Approach this as a joint venture, where both partners contribute equally to restore and enhance their intimacy.

It's essential not to underestimate the power of apologies and forgiveness in this process. Imperfect communication is inevitable. Missteps will happen, and feelings will sometimes get hurt. The willingness to apologise sincerely and offer forgiveness is a testament to the strength and resilience of your relationship. These actions remind both partners of their humanity and shared commitment to moving forward together, reinforcing the safety and strength of the space you are creating.

Fostering a safe space for communication also requires patience. Change rarely comes overnight. As both partners adjust to this new way of communicating, patience and persistence are required. Encourage each other, celebrate small victories, and remain committed to the process. In doing so, you'll find that obstacles become easier to overcome, and discussions about difficult topics, like issues of sexual desire, become less daunting.

In sum, creating a safe space for communication isn't just about solving problems—it's about fortifying your relationship, nurturing trust, and ensuring both partners feel valued and understood. By putting these principles into practice, you're not only addressing current issues but also establishing a strong foundation for navigating future challenges together. The journey towards deeper, more open communication could become one of the most rewarding aspects of your relationship, ultimately leading to a more fulfilling and passionate connection.

## Overcoming Shame and Stigma

In the journey of restoring intimacy and passion, shame and stigma can be significant hurdles. These feelings are not always openly discussed, yet they quietly persist, hindering men from embracing and addressing their struggles with libido loss. Recognising and overcoming these barriers is essential for engaging in open dialogue with themselves and their partners. This section explores how shame and stigma manifest and offers strategies to transcend them.

Shame often arises from societal expectations of masculinity and sexual performance. Many men have grown up with the notion that their worth is tied to their sexual prowess, and any deviation from this expectation can lead to feelings of inadequacy. Society's portrayal of men as always eager and ready for sexual encounters contributes to this pressure. If a man's libido wanes, he may worry about being perceived as less of a man, which can prevent him from openly discussing these changes.

Moreover, stigma surrounding men's sexual health issues can be particularly corrosive. Discussing libido loss is not a common practice among male peers. This silence feeds into the perception that a decrease in sexual desire is abnormal or embarrassing, reinforcing the idea that it should be kept hidden. Breaking the cycle of silence requires courage, but it's a crucial step towards healing and growth. The support of partners and a community that encourages openness can significantly help dismantle these stigmas.

It's important to understand that acknowledging a decline in libido is not an admission of failure. It is, rather, recognition of a natural and sometimes transient phase of life that many men experience. Normalising these changes is key to reducing the stigma attached. Partners, too, play a vital role in this process. By adopting an empathetic and understanding approach, they help create a safe environment that encourages open communication.

Open dialogue involves more than just speaking out; it requires listening and being truly present. Listening without judgement allows individuals to express themselves freely, which can relieve them from the burden of shame. This active listening helps partners understand that libido issues do not diminish affection or the potential for a fulfilling relationship. It is a team effort, where both partners can explore strategies and solutions together.

The role of partners in dispelling shame cannot be overstated. They can initiate conversations that reassure the other that a decrease in sexual desire doesn't equate to a lack of love or attraction. It also helps to focus on the emotional aspects of the relationship, emphasising the importance of intimacy beyond physical intercourse. This shift in focus can alleviate some of the pressure tied to performance, allowing for a more relaxed and open dynamic between partners.

Meanwhile, individual introspection is equally vital. Self-compassion is a powerful tool in overcoming shame. Recognising one's worth beyond sexual performance and embracing vulnerabilities are key to this process. Men should remind themselves of their unique qualities and contributions that extend beyond sexuality. Engaging in practices such as mindfulness or journaling can support this self-reflection, offering insights into feelings and behaviours connected to libido.

Education plays a critical role in overcoming stigma. By understanding the numerous psychological, physical, and relational factors influencing libido, men can view their experiences not as isolated incidents but as part of a broader, more complex picture. This understanding can break down the misconceptions that contribute to feelings of shame, replacing them with a more informed and positive perspective.

Communities and support networks provide additional avenues for overcoming stigma. Men's groups and forums focused on sexual health can offer an anonymous yet supportive space for men to share experiences and solutions. These platforms can be instrumental in normalising conversations around libido, as they affirm that many men face similar challenges and that sharing is not only acceptable but beneficial.

Building a partnership where both individuals feel open and unburdened by shame is an ongoing process. It involves regular check-ins, honest conversations, and mutual respect for each other's experiences and feelings. By fostering a culture of transparency, couples can bolster their relationship's resilience, allowing them to weather not only issues related to libido but other significant challenges as well.

Men who actively engage in overcoming shame and stigma may find a renewed sense of self-esteem and agency. They realise that seeking help and discussing their feelings are not signs of weakness but of strength. Every step taken towards openness strengthens their intimate connections and personal well-being.

Together, as partners and individuals, men can navigate the landscape of libido challenges with a newfound liberation from shame and stigma. This journey is one of growth, understanding, and continual evolution, ultimately aiming to redefine what it means to have a fulfilling and intimate relationship.

## Listening Skills and Feedback

Effective listening is more than just the act of hearing words. It's about fully immersing oneself in the conversation, understanding underlying emotions, and cultivating an environment where partners feel valued and heard. In the context of declining sexual desire, good listening skills are pivotal for rebuilding intimacy and trust. When one partner listens genuinely, it signals that they're invested in understanding their partner's experiences and emotions.

Engaging in open dialogue without the barriers of judgment or preconceived notions allows for more honest and meaningful exchanges. It's crucial that both partners approach discussions with a mindset of empathy and curiosity rather than criticism or defence. This means consciously silencing that inner voice that might jump to conclusions or assumptions. When we truly listen, we validate our partner's feelings, even if we don't agree with them, thus strengthening the emotional bond.

An essential aspect of listening involves giving feedback that reflects understanding and empathy. Feedback isn't about offering solutions or immediately trying to "fix" a situation. Oftentimes, your partner might just want to feel seen and understood. Active listening facilitates this by allowing pauses in the conversation where thoughts can be gathered, and emotions processed. During these moments, nodding or gentle affirmations like "I understand" or "That sounds difficult" foster a sense of solidarity.

Listening, especially in emotionally charged discussions, requires one to manage their own emotional responses. Practising deep listening means resisting the urge to interrupt or defend oneself. It's about allowing the speaker to express themselves fully, which can be challenging if what they are saying triggers a defensive response. By practising patience and maintaining a calm and supportive demeanour, partners can ensure that conversations remain constructive and focused on understanding rather than winning an argument.

Offering feedback should come from a place of support and care. It's helpful to use "I" statements, like "I feel" or "I think", to express how the conversation affects you without coming across as accusatory. For instance, instead of saying, "You never consider how I feel," try, "I feel unheard when our conversations focus only on solutions without acknowledging the emotions involved." This approach helps maintain a balanced and fair dialogue, where both partners' perspectives are equally valued.

Additionally, it's crucial to be mindful of non-verbal cues. Body language can either reinforce or undermine the spoken word. Maintaining eye contact, nodding, or leaning slightly forward signals engagement and attentiveness. Conversely, crossed arms, distracted gazes, or sighing can convey disinterest, even if unintentionally. Awareness of these signals ensures that non-verbal communication aligns with one's words.

Encouraging open dialogue requires creating a safe space where vulnerability is protected, and each person feels supported. This space allows for reflection and growth, where partners can express fears, desires, and concerns without fear of invalidation or ridicule. Setting boundaries about what is and isn't okay—constructive criticism, not personal attacks, for instance—can enhance this safe space.

Listening well reaffirms the value of the relationship. It helps dismantle barriers of resentment and misunderstanding, paving the way for a renewed connection. When both partners commit to practicing active listening and providing thoughtful feedback, the relationship can move from a place of conflict or apathy towards a revitalised and more connected state.

Often, partners may struggle with staying present in a conversation, especially when the issues discussed are complex or emotionally loaded. Mindfulness can serve as a powerful tool for enhancing listening skills. By focusing on the present moment and gently releasing distracting thoughts, partners can better engage with the conversation at hand. This not only benefits the listener but can help the speaker feel more at ease and open.

The path to mastering listening skills and providing constructive feedback might be riddled with occasional missteps. Perhaps a harsh word slips out or a defensive posture is taken; it's important to view these instances as learning opportunities. Each mistake carries the potential for growth. When they occur, addressing them candidly, with the acknowledgment of one's errors, helps renew trust and demonstrates commitment to improving the dialogue.

Furthermore, understanding and utilising these listening skills in tandem with receiving feedback requires patience and practice. Relationships, especially those weathering the challenges of declining sexual desire, benefit immensely from such dedication to communication. The fruits of this labour are a relationship buoyed by mutual understanding and a rekindled intimacy that acknowledges and respects both partners' needs and stories.

Incorporating listening as a deliberate practice in everyday conversations strengthens relationships beyond the realm of sexuality. It cultivates an environment in which both partners feel equipped to express themselves openly and without reservation, ushering in a newfound closeness. This lays the groundwork for tackling more profound issues and exploring solutions, not in isolation, but together as a united front.

To cultivate effective listening skills, partners might consider regular check-ins or "listening moments" during the week, providing dedicated time where each person has the floor to share freely without interruption. Setting aside this time emphasizes the value placed on open dialogue and can become a cherished ritual that fosters continual connection and understanding.

Practise active listening by focusing entirely on your partner when they speak.

Avoid preparing your response while the other is talking; instead, absorb what is being communicated.

Use feedback as a means to reflect understanding, employing empathetic language.

Be mindful of non-verbal communication and its potential impact on the dialogue.

Address and learn from any communication missteps, reinforcing the relationship's resilience.

Ultimately, listening is an art that, when honed with intention and care, opens doors to more meaningful connections and pathways to deeper emotional and physical intimacy. As practice cultivates these skills, they become integral to the fabric of the relationship, woven into every conversation and shared decision, sustaining a partnership rich in understanding and love.

# Chapter 23:
## Designing Personalised Action Plans

Crafting a personalised action plan is an empowering step towards revitalising intimacy and addressing the unique challenges of libido loss. It's essential to set realistic, achievable goals that reflect personal desires and circumstances, creating a tailored roadmap that aligns with one's life and relationship dynamics. Begin by identifying specific areas for improvement, such as enhancing communication with your partner or integrating mindfulness practices into daily routines. As you embark on this journey, keep track of your progress and celebrate each success, no matter how small. This not only bolsters motivation, but it also provides a sense of accomplishment that fuels ongoing efforts. Remember, flexibility is key; be prepared to adapt strategies as your needs evolve. At the core of this approach is understanding that every individual's path is distinct, and by honouring personal stories and experiences, a truly meaningful transformation is possible. Embrace this opportunity for growth, keeping in mind that it's as much about the journey as it is about the destination—enhancing your connection, confidence, and ultimately reigniting passion in your relationship.

## Setting Realistic Goals

Designing personalised action plans to rekindle intimacy requires more than just a broad set of guidelines—it demands the crafting of goals that are both attainable and meaningful. Essential to this process is the

197

understanding that realistic goals serve as stepping stones toward the larger objective of rejuvenating a diminishing libido and enhancing intimate relationships. So, how do we establish these goals without the overhang of unrealistic expectations?

First, it's critical to begin with a self-assessment. Reflect on the aspects of your relationship that you hold dear and identify areas where you sense a void. Are there specific moments or encounters where your interest tends to wane? Understanding these nuances can illuminate the path toward setting targets that directly address the issues at hand. This requires honesty and a willingness to confront truths that may be uncomfortable but ultimately necessary for progress.

It's beneficial to employ the SMART criteria—Specific, Measurable, Achievable, Relevant, and Time-bound—when crafting goals. Specificity sharpens the focus, making each goal more tangible. Instead of a nebulous aim like "improve intimacy," set a goal such as "increase meaningful conversations with my partner each week." Such a target is not only clear but also actionable.

Measuring progress is vital for motivation and course correction. Regular check-ins, perhaps weekly or fortnightly, can provide tangible insights into your advancement. This practice isn't about criticising shortcomings but celebrating progress and recalibrating when necessary. For example, if a goal is to explore new date night activities once a month, you can track which activities truly elevate the relational experience and which ones miss the mark.

Achievability relates directly to setting a pace that respects your capabilities and limits. Goals that stretch too far too quickly can lead to frustration rather than fulfilment. That's why it's crucial to balance aspiration with realism. Start with smaller, immediately achievable steps to build momentum. For instance, if your current routine allows for very little downtime together, aim first for adding a weekly hour of undistracted time before attempting more elaborate engagements.

The relevance of a goal serves as a reminder that each objective should resonate with both partners' values and desires. A goal ought to be mutually beneficial to ensure both parties feel invested. If intimacy issues stem from a lack of shared activities, picking a new hobby together can be both relevant and rewarding.

Timelines should guide rather than pressure. Set an overarching timeframe that maintains your focus while allowing for flexibility. Life undoubtedly introduces disruptions and surprises; maintaining some elasticity in timing can prevent unnecessary stress and keep morale high. For instance, if you aim to heighten your sexual confidence, let this goal span six months rather than weeks, providing ample room for gradual change.

Beyond constructing goals, envisioning the end result can be immensely powerful. Visualisation techniques can play a role in manifesting the aspirations you're working towards. Imagine how fulfilling it will be when you've achieved the intimacy level you yearn for. These mental exercises not only cook motivation but also clarify which paths will lead most directly to your destinations.

At times, external input can refine your goals into even clearer focus. Consulting a couples' therapist or a relationship counsellor can offer perspective and guidance, ensuring your goals remain aligned with healthy relationship dynamics. These professionals can provide feedback rooted in experience and knowledge, sometimes illuminating blind spots you didn't know existed.

Although this journey is deeply personal, involving your partner in the goal-setting process can transform it into a shared expedition. A joint approach to these goals fosters communication and cooperation, turning what might have been an individual struggle into a collaborative effort. Discussions about each other's needs, boundaries, and desires can refine the direction and nature of your goals.

Tracking progress and acknowledging small victories along the way can exponentially increase commitment to the process. Celebrations, whether they involve a special night out or a simple acknowledgment, reinforce positive behaviours and alleviate some of the pressures of a long-term endeavour. Even a simple "we did it!" can lift spirits and encourage further commitment.

Developing a feedback loop enriches the process, providing time to reflect on what works and what doesn't. It's important not to self-criticise when goals aren't met as planned; instead, view each setback as a stepping stone towards deeper understanding and eventual success. Adjusting and refining goals is not a sign of failure but a testament to growth and learning.

Ultimately, setting realistic goals in the context of a declining libido requires both introspection and interaction. It's a delicate balance that hinges on patience, openness, and a willingness to adapt. The path may be fraught with challenges, but it also promises the profound reward of a revitalised connection. With purpose and perseverance, these goals can pave the way to a reawakened intimacy that affirms the depth and resilience of the relationship.

## Tracking Progress and Celebrating Success

Embarking on the journey to revitalise sexual desire and intimacy is akin to crafting a beautiful tapestry, where each thread represents individual efforts, breakthroughs, and moments of growth. Within this transformative process, tracking progress becomes an essential practice—one that not only provides insight into what's working but also keeps motivation alive. By identifying and acknowledging the small victories along the way, one cultivates a sense of accomplishment that paves the way for larger successes.

It's crucial to remember that progress doesn't always happen at a steady pace. There will be phases of rapid advancement interspersed with periods of slower change. These fluctuations are normal and should be anticipated. By setting realistic benchmarks and continually assessing the journey, you can maintain a clear vision of where you're headed, adjusting strategies as needed without losing sight of the ultimate goal: reigniting passion and building a stronger relationship.

Begin by defining what success looks like for you and your partner. What are the signs that indicate improvement? Perhaps it's increased openness in communication or a newfound enthusiasm for shared activities. Whatever the indicators, make sure they're personal and meaningful. Having clear objectives not only provides a roadmap but also offers tangible evidence of growth when those objectives are met. Additionally, breaking down these goals into smaller, manageable steps can help in maintaining focus and momentum.

Regular check-ins are invaluable when tracking progress. Setting aside dedicated time to reflect on achievements—no matter how minor they may seem—reinforces positive behaviour and encourages continued effort. Consider using a journal to note down significant moments or changes in perception. Recording experiences not only tracks growth but also acts as a reminder of the journey undertaken.

Furthermore, celebrating success plays a critical role in sustaining motivation. It's a means of acknowledging the hard work put into the process and serves as a reward system that reinforces positive actions. Celebrations don't need to be grand gestures; they could be as simple as a quiet dinner, a day out, or even just words of affirmation and encouragement exchanged between partners. These acts of celebration help to solidify the progress made and inject a sense of joy and accomplishment into the journey.

Incorporating flexibility into your action plan is also essential. Life is unpredictable, and unforeseen circumstances or setbacks can occur. When faced with obstacles, it's important to revisit the original objectives and assess whether they need adaptation. Doing so doesn't signify failure but demonstrates resilience and an ability to overcome challenges. Adaptability ensures that the action plan remains relevant and attainable, no matter what complications arise.

There's a psychological boost that comes with recognising progress. Just as you track improvements in other areas of health—like fitness or nutrition—being aware of developments in sexual health can create a positive feedback loop. This heightened awareness fosters a stronger connection to one's physical and emotional state, adding depth and meaning to the experiences shared with a partner.

Sharing successes with your partner is integral to reinforcing the foundations of your relationship. Expressing gratitude for each other's efforts, identifying how the changes have positively impacted your dynamic, and discussing future aspirations fosters an atmosphere of teamwork and unity. These discussions can lead to an enhanced understanding and greater emotional closeness, which further stokes the flame of intimacy.

Moreover, the act of celebrating achievements cultivates an optimistic mindset that's fuelled by hope and enthusiasm. This shift in perspective is powerful—it encourages a perception that change is not only possible but attainable and significant. Embracing this mindset can transform your approach to challenges, promoting a sense of empowerment and self-efficacy.

As progress is made, it's also important to recalibrate expectations as necessary. Understanding that not every goal will be reached in the anticipated timeframe can prevent disillusionment. By acknowledging that this journey is uniquely personal and non-linear, you can reduce pressure and foster a more nurturing environment for growth.

Lastly, remember that documenting and celebrating progress sends a profound message: that the journey towards rekindling intimacy is valuable and worth cherishing. Each step, regardless of its size, contributes to a resilient and thriving relationship enriched by understanding, empathy, and love. Celebrate the journey as much as the destination, and take solace in knowing these efforts are reshaping your intimate partnership for the better.

## Adapting Strategies to Fit Individual Needs

In the journey towards revitalising one's libido and enhancing intimate relationships, personalised action plans are crucial. It's not just about following generic advice; it's about tailoring strategies that resonate with your needs and lifestyle. The essence of personalisation lies in its flexibility, allowing individuals to adapt and refine approaches as they navigate through their unique circumstances. Understanding this is an empowering step, making the process not only effective but also deeply personal.

Consider the diverse backdrop of experiences and challenges that can influence one's sexual desire. From physical health variations to differing psychological landscapes, each person's situation demands a nuanced approach. It's here where adaptability becomes indispensable. The same strategy that works wonders for one individual might fall flat for another, underscoring the need for a bespoke approach. Therefore, the understanding that strategies should evolve as life circumstances and needs change is key.

Implementing and experimenting with different approaches can be a revelatory experience. It starts with a willingness to acknowledge what has worked for you in the past and what hasn't. This involves a degree of introspection and honesty that can be challenging but rewarding. By assessing your unique triggers and desires, you can begin to craft a strategy tailored specifically to reignite your passion. For instance, you may find that physical exercise plays a significant role in your sexual health, necessitating a focus on routines that enhance physical vitality.

Next, let's talk about the vital role of communication in personalising your action plan. Open dialogue with your partner is indispensable when adapting strategies to individual needs. Engaging in honest conversations about desires, preferences, and boundaries can shed light on areas that require attention. This collaborative approach not only strengthens the bond between partners but also ensures that the strategies you're adopting are feasible and mutually beneficial.

Flexibility is another critical component of adapting strategies. Life is full of unpredictable changes, whether they're related to stress, health, or external commitments. Therefore, it's crucial to allow adjustments in your plan as these changes arise. This might involve temporarily prioritising mental health strategies if stress becomes overwhelming, or perhaps focusing on physical health when confronted with lifestyle-related illnesses. Whatever the case, adaptability ensures that the focus remains on long-term success.

Furthermore, in the quest to adapt strategies, embracing a growth mindset is instrumental. Viewing challenges as opportunities for growth can transform setbacks into valuable learning experiences. It's about fostering resilience and using each experience, whether successful or not, as a stepping stone to better understanding your personal needs and goals. This mindset not only aids in overcoming present challenges but also equips you with a robust framework for future obstacles.

Additionally, tracking progress is a facet of personalisation that can't be overlooked. After establishing tailored strategies, it's important to monitor and evaluate their effectiveness regularly. This not only helps in identifying areas that may require further refinement but also serves to celebrate the victories, no matter how small. Progress tracking involves setting benchmarks and goals that are aligned with your capabilities, ensuring that each goal feels attainable and relevant to your journey.

In parallel, cultural factors also play a significant role in shaping individual strategies. Cultural backgrounds can influence expectations, beliefs, and practices related to sexuality, necessitating an approach that's sensitive to these aspects. Awareness and respect for cultural differences ensure that the strategies adopted are not only practical but also respectful and inclusive, fostering a supportive environment in which positive change can occur.

Let's also delve into the importance of seeking professional guidance when needed. Sometimes, tailoring a strategy to fit your individual needs can benefit from expert insight. Therapists, counsellors, or sexual health professionals can offer a treasure trove of personalised advice and techniques that align with your circumstances. This also helps in unearthing underlying issues that might require more focused attention, whether through therapy sessions or specialised interventions.

But what about the weight of societal norms and expectations? These too can define how one approaches sexual health and intimacy. Reflecting on and perhaps challenging these norms can lead to a profound realignment of personal strategies. For instance, shedding the pressure to conform to certain stereotypes about male sexuality allows one to pursue a more genuine, individualized path towards reawakening desire.

The journey towards reigniting passion shouldn't be undertaken in isolation. The involvement of a partner not only enriches the experience but ensures that strategies align with shared goals and expectations. It's a symbiotic dance of understanding, where both partners feel valued and heard, paving the way for a more fulfilling intimate life.

Ultimately, adapting strategies to fit individual needs is about crafting a blueprint that's ever-evolving. It's a tapestry woven with understanding, introspection, and flexibility. By embracing the idiosyncrasies of personal experiences and challenges, individuals can chart a course that not only enhances their intimate relationships but also enriches their overall quality of life. With a steadfast commitment to personal growth and a readiness to adapt, the journey to reigniting lost desire transforms from a daunting task into an empowering adventure.

# Chapter 24:
# The Impact of Technology and Media

As we delve into the realms of technology and media, it's essential to acknowledge how profoundly they shape our perceptions, especially concerning intimacy and libido. The digital age offers a dizzying array of information and stimuli, often depicting exaggerated ideals of sexuality that can distort our expectations and self-image. This landscape, albeit filled with valuable insights, requires mindful navigation to prevent its adverse effects on personal relationships and one's sense of self-worth. Through conscious moderation of content consumption, individuals and couples can foster a healthy balance that prioritizes genuine connection over fleeting digital interactions. Ethical considerations should guide our engagement with media, prompting discussions about authenticity and self-reflection. By harnessing technology as a tool for enhancement rather than comparison, we can protect and nurture our intimate relationships, paving the way for meaningful and lasting fulfilment.

## Media's Influence on Perceptions

In today's interconnected world, technology and media wield substantial power over our perceptions. They craft narratives, influence beliefs, and shape ideas about almost every facet of life, including sexuality and intimacy. The portrayal of male sexuality in media can act as both an informer and a distorter, impacting how men perceive their own sexual desires and capabilities. While media can provide valuable insights and expand knowledge, it also bears the risk of perpetuating unrealistic standards and misconceptions about libido, which can contribute to personal dissatisfaction and relationship challenges.

Consider the prevalence of hypersexualised content in media. Films, TV shows, and advertisements often depict men with inexhaustible sexual desires, brimming with confidence and skill. These depictions can lead to an internalised misunderstanding about how 'normal' libido should manifest. For many men, such portrayals establish an unachievable benchmark, pushing them to measure their own experiences against a fictional standard. This often results in feelings of inadequacy and frustration when their reality doesn't match up with the media-created image. This tension can further exacerbate libido issues, creating a cycle of self-doubt.

Moreover, the concept of masculinity portrayed through media can be heavily influenced by stereotypes that equate male worth with sexual prowess. When media bombards individuals with such associations, it enforces a narrow view that diminishes the complexities of male sexuality. Instead of embracing a broad spectrum of desires and personal circumstances, men might find themselves pressured to prove their masculinity in ways that overlook emotional depth and vulnerability. This can deter open communication with partners and create a barrier to seeking help when experiencing libido declines.

It's not just traditional media that's in play. Social media platforms now offer an endless feed of 'advice', testimonials, and assumptions about what constitutes a healthy sex life. Amidst influencers and self-proclaimed experts, distinguishing between factual content and opinion becomes challenging. Men may come across seemingly straightforward solutions to libido issues scattered across blogs and vlogs. However, many of these suggestions lack the nuance necessary to address underlying issues, offering placebo-like reassurance rather than practical help.

On the other hand, the media can also play a positive role by providing a platform for diverse narratives and expert voices. Documentaries, podcasts, and articles featuring medical professionals or sex therapists can offer enlightening perspectives that counterbalance the simplistic ways in which masculinity and libido are often portrayed. These resources can educate men, helping them understand that experiencing fluctuations in libido is a normal part of human life, and not inherently indicative of a deeper problem.

For partners and individuals seeking to reignite intimacy in their relationships, being conscious of media's influence is crucial. Critically assessing the content they consume can enhance their self-awareness, allowing them to better separate media-induced perceptions from their authentic experiences and desires. Partners should discuss and reflect on how media influence each of them, opening a dialogue that can lead to more grounded expectations and healing connections.

As media continues to evolve, it's essential to actively curate one's media landscape. Opting for varied sources and seeking content by trusted professionals can mitigate the risk of misconceptions. Additionally, practising digital mindfulness by setting boundaries on media consumption can nurture mental health and reinforce positive self-images. The ability to discern beneficial information from media noise becomes a vital skill for those navigating personal relationships and sexual health.

Looking broader, the conversation about media influence on perceptions begs a cultural shift in framing masculinity and sexuality. Society benefits from media that embraces diversity in experiences and narratives, moving away from clichés toward more inclusive representations. Initiatives encouraging media literacy should be supported, fostering a critical understanding among audiences about the impact of what they consume.

Ultimately, as long as media maintains its powerful hold on societal perceptions, awareness and education remain key. Men and their partners embarking on a path to reclaim libido and rekindle intimacy should strive for a balance between gaining insights from media and nurturing an authentic appreciation for their unique experiences. By doing so, they take tangible steps toward reshaping the narrative around male sexuality, embracing both its challenges and its joys. Embracing this journey with open hearts and minds transforms perceived deficits into opportunities for connection and growth.

## Moderating Content Consumption

In the cacophony of modern life, technology and media surround us with ceaseless chatter. They promise connection and entertainment, yet often obscure the delicate balance of intimacy. It's easy for content consumption to become excessive, affecting perceptions and skewing our views on relationships and self-worth. Understanding how to moderate these influences can be a pivotal step in addressing declines in sexual desire and enhancing personal connections.

The advent of technology allows for constant access to information and entertainment, transforming the way we consume media. This seamless availability comes with its own set of challenges, particularly in affecting how we perceive relationships and sexuality. When bombarded with unrealistic portrayals of intimacy, it's easy to internalise a distorted view of what sexual and emotional connection should look like. This, in turn, can lead to feelings of inadequacy or dissatisfaction with one's own sex life.

What we consume affects our cognitive processes. Engaging in a diet of sensationalised or exaggerated accounts of romance and physical attractiveness can create unrealistic benchmarks. Men experiencing a decrease in libido may feel pressure from these distorted standards, which can exacerbate feelings of inadequacy. It is crucial to recognise these pressures, understand their roots, and develop strategies to guard against them.

Finding balance in content consumption starts with awareness. Acknowledging the types of media that might negatively impact your view on relationships is the first step. With this awareness comes the ability to make conscious choices about what content you engage with. The goal is to choose media that uplifts and informs, rather than content that might diminish self-esteem or create unrealistic expectations.

Intentional media consumption can shift perspectives and rekindle the spark of desire. Curating content that speaks to personal values and realistic portrayals of intimacy can act as a motivational and enlightening tool. This involves seeking out narratives that emphasise authenticity, communication, and mutual respect in relationships. By doing so, it encourages a healthier view of one's own experiences and expectations.

Moreover, creating boundaries around content consumption is essential. Set specific times to engage with media and stick to them. This practice not only limits exposure to potentially detrimental content but also frees up time for self-reflection and interaction with one's partner. Being present in your relationship often means being less present online.

Digital detoxification can rejuvenate the mind and body. Consider instituting technology-free zones within the household or technology-free times during the day, particularly during shared activities. This conscious disconnection helps nurture emotional closeness and provides space for genuine interaction. In creating space for deeper connection away from screens, couples may find it easier to explore and address issues affecting their intimacy.

In addition, discussing media consumption with your partner can be an enlightening exercise. Open discussions about how media messages relate to personal experiences help both partners understand each other's viewpoints and reinforce shared values. Collaborative reflection on media exposure also fosters empathy, enabling partners to support each other in reinforcing positive messages and negating harmful stereotypes.

While media portrays idealised forms of sexual engagement, it's crucial to remember that every relationship is unique and thrives on personal input rather than scripted perfection. Emphasising this individuality can help relieve any pressure stemming from external portrayals of ideal intimacy. Sharing these insights with your partner can support a journey together to reinforce a shared reality.

Ultimately, assertive moderation of content consumption serves not just to shield oneself from negative influences but to enrich the relationship with informed and empathetic viewpoints. By choosing nutritious content and consuming mindfully, you're not just improving an understanding of intimate dynamics but also investing in the quality and depth of your relationships.

As we navigate the digital age, let moderation be an ally in rekindling passion and understanding. An intentional approach to media consumption, balanced with genuine connection, enriches every aspect of life, emphasising the beauty in subtleties and authenticity in relationships. By taking control of what influences us, it's possible to forge stronger bonds, build self-esteem, and ignite the fully nourished desire that feels just as it should.

## Ethical Considerations and Balance

In a world increasingly saturated with technology and media, navigating the landscape of digital influences presents not only possibilities but profound challenges, particularly in the sphere of intimacy and relationships. The potential for technology to enhance communication and provide educational resources is undeniable. However, it also requires ethical considerations to ensure these tools are used wisely, without undermining personal relationships or distorting perceptions of intimacy.

At the heart of the ethical debate is the ubiquitous nature of media portrayals that often suggest skewed ideals and expectations. While these can serve as inspiration for some, they can just as easily create unrealistic benchmarks for others, potentially leading to dissatisfaction or self-doubt. It's critical to recognise that media representations—be they of relationships, body image, or sexual prowess—are often idealised and may not reflect the complexities and imperfections of real life.

As individuals grappling with changes in libido or desire, it becomes imperative to distinguish between idealised media narratives and personal truths. The first step is cultivating awareness. Are the media and technological platforms you engage with enhancing your understanding and connection with your partner, or are they driving a wedge by fostering unattainable ideals? Developing media literacy—an ability to critically evaluate the content consumed—can empower individuals to make discerning choices about the information they incorporate into their lives.

Consider the impact of social media, a digital force that has shaped modern perceptions in ways previously unimaginable. On platforms where life is curated, the reality of fluctuating desires within a relationship is often hidden. This can feed into feelings of inadequacy or failure, especially in intimate settings. Couples might find themselves comparing their relationship to the highlight reels of others, which rarely, if ever, display the full picture. It's vital to maintain a balanced perception, where self-worth and relationship health are not dictated by virtual validation but by genuine connection and understanding.

Moreover, the ethics of privacy and consent are crucial when engaging with technology in the context of intimacy. Couples may choose to incorporate digital tools to spice things up, such as through intimate texts, shared playlists, or perhaps exciting wearables. Yet, there must be a mutual understanding and respect for boundaries. Decisions to utilise or share digital content should always be consensual, safeguarding personal privacy and trust.

Technology, when wielded responsibly, offers boundless opportunities for learning and enhancing relationships. Online platforms can provide access to expert insights, fostering knowledge that empowers individuals in their journey to rekindle intimacy. However, this accessibility comes with the responsibility of filtering through misinformation. Not every source professing to hold the keys to a happier relationship bears credibility. Individuals and couples must strive to seek information from reputable, ethical sources that value scientific evidence and professional integrity.

Balance is an ongoing theme in ethical considerations regarding technology and media. Balance involves moderation in content consumption, ensuring time spent online does not eclipse time spent nurturing real-world relationships. It is about finding a sweet spot where technology serves as a beneficial adjunct to, rather than a replacement for, genuine interaction and exploration of intimacy.

Practically, achieving this balance could mean setting boundaries around technology use. Establishing tech-free times, particularly during shared moments of intimacy or important discussions, allows partners to connect without distractions. Creating an environment that prioritises face-to-face engagement reinforces a culture of presence and attentiveness, critical components of strong relationships.

In conclusion, there's a delicate interplay between the influence of technology and media and the very personal domain of sexual desire and intimacy. By approaching this interplay with an ethical mindset, individuals and couples can navigate their paths more consciously, making decisions that uplift rather than diminish the sacredness of their relationships. The key lies in thoughtful engagement with technology—harnessing its benefits while remaining vigilant about its pitfalls, always keeping focus on maintaining healthy, realistic, and truly human connections.

# Chapter 25:
## Sustainable Habits for Long-Term Success

Maintaining a fulfilling and intimate relationship over time isn't just about quick fixes or grand gestures; rather, it's carved from the consistency of sustainable habits. Developing routines that you and your partner can rely on, like regular times to connect emotionally and physically, grounds your relationship in trust and intimacy. Focusing on small, manageable changes can sometimes yield the most meaningful shifts. Perhaps it's about dedicating a few minutes each day to truly listen to each other's needs, or embarking on a shared hobby that brings laughter and connection. Motivation can ebb and flow, but nurturing these habits with patience and persistence can embody the commitment to a healthier, more passionate partnership. This isn't about perfection, but rather about progress and the shared journey towards deepened bonds and lasting harmony.

## Developing Consistent Routines

Developing consistent routines is the cornerstone of sustainable habits for long-term success, particularly when confronting a decline in sexual desire. Establishing a routine that supports your overall health and well-being can have a profound impact on your libido and intimate relationships. Often, it's the small, incremental changes that lead to the most significant results. While daunting at first, consistent routines eventually transform into natural elements of daily life, promoting a stable environment for both personal growth and relationship enhancement.

One of the first steps in developing a consistent routine is identifying patterns that already exist in your life. Consider your daily habits, from how you start your day to the way you prepare for sleep. By pinpointing these automatic behaviours, you can determine which ones serve your goals and which may need adjustment. For instance, integrating a morning stretch or walk can invigorate your senses and contribute positively to your physical health, setting a productive tone for the day.

Achieving consistency requires both intentionality and flexibility. While laying down a regimented plan can be helpful, it's equally important to remain adaptable to life's unpredictability. Whether it's a family commitment or an unplanned work obligation, disruptions occur. By cultivating an adaptable mindset, you allow room for flexibility without losing sight of your routine's core objectives. This flexibility helps maintain progress without feeling hindered by perfectionism.

When it comes to revitalising libido specifically, routines around diet, exercise, and mindfulness play pivotal roles. Regular exercise not only boosts physical fitness but also enhances mood and stress levels, crucial factors in sexual health. Engaging in physical activity consistently is shown to promote the release of endorphins and increase testosterone levels, thereby positively influencing libido. Finding an activity you enjoy ensures it becomes a sustainable part of your life rather than a chore you dread.

Diet, too, can be woven into a consistent routine. Simple dietary changes, such as prioritising whole foods over processed options and staying hydrated, offer long-term benefits. Planning meals and snacks can prevent last-minute unhealthy choices and foster a balanced approach to nutrition. Additionally, staying mindful of alcohol and caffeine intake can stabilise energy levels and mood, further supporting a healthy libido.

Creating routines around mindfulness and mental health can contribute significantly to managing stress and anxiety—common inhibitors of sexual desire. Incorporating techniques like meditation, deep breathing, or even journaling into your daily schedule encourages self-awareness and emotional regulation. These practices offer a moment of introspection and calm in an often chaotic world, enabling you to approach intimate relationships from a place of tranquillity and presence.

Beyond individual practices, sharing and communicating your routines with your partner can strengthen your relationship. Engaging in joint activities, like cooking a meal together or participating in a fitness class, fosters a sense of connection and mutual support. Developing shared rituals doesn't just boost your libido; it reinforces trust and emotional intimacy, key components in a fulfilling relationship.

The initial transition to new routines can be challenging. It's common to face resistance or struggle with motivation, but the secret lies in perseverance and celebrating small victories. Remember, growth isn't linear, and setbacks don't equate to failure. By focusing on progress over perfection and viewing each day as an opportunity to recommit, routines gradually transform into an integral part of your lifestyle.

Moreover, evaluating the effectiveness of your routines regularly ensures they remain aligned with your changing needs and circumstances. Reflection allows you to determine what's working, what's not, and where adjustments might be necessary. It's a practice of mindfulness in itself, encouraging continual growth and improvement without judgement or criticism.

In developing these consistent routines, it helps to enlist support where needed. Whether through professional guidance or a community of like-minded individuals, sharing the journey can offer encouragement and accountability. Understanding you're not alone in your efforts reduces feelings of isolation and enhances motivation to maintain these positive changes.

Finally, integrating consistent routines into your life doesn't mean being rigid or uncompromising. It's about crafting a balanced approach that aligns with your values and life aspirations while accommodating the ebbs and flows of daily life. By weaving together the threads of healthy diet, regular physical activity, mental wellness practices, and nurturing relationship habits, you create a tapestry of habits that supports long-term success in both personal well-being and intimate relationships.

Building sustainable habits takes time and effort, but the rewards—a rejuvenated libido, strengthened partnerships, and overall improved quality of life—are well worth the investment. As you establish these routines, you'll find that the journey towards reviving intimacy and enhancing your relationship becomes not just a goal, but a path you tread together, fostering deeper understanding and connection with both yourself and your partner.

## Emphasising Small Changes

Breaking down overwhelming challenges into manageable parts is often the key to success in many aspects of life, including reigniting passion and enhancing intimate relationships. When faced with a decline in sexual desire, the thought of overhauling your lifestyle or relationship dynamic can feel daunting. But here's where small changes come into play. They're the humble yet powerful steps that lay the foundation for sustainable change without inducing stress or pressure.

Picture the growth of a tree: a seed doesn't transform into a towering oak overnight. Instead, it takes root, gradually expanding over time. Similarly, small adjustments in lifestyle, health habits, and interpersonal communication serve as the seeds that foster enhanced libido and relationship satisfaction. Start by embracing these minor modifications not as mundane chores, but as exciting opportunities for growth and self-discovery. This perspective shift is vital for maintaining motivation and commitment over the long haul.

The power of small changes is well-illustrated by habit-forming techniques. Consider embracing a new routine; these changes don't demand immediate perfection. They encourage you to build consistent and healthy habits at a comfortable pace. For instance, incorporating a brief daily meditation practice can enhance your mindfulness, ultimately leading to a more profound connection with both yourself and your partner. Over time, this single step can significantly impact emotional intimacy and sexual desire.

Start with something as simple as open communication. Set aside five minutes each day to check in with your partner, discussing the highs and lows of your day. This practice might seem minor, but it fosters emotional closeness and understanding, both crucial elements in reviving passion. Instead of focusing on reaching an immediate outcome, take pride in committing to this dialogue, knowing it's nurturing your relationship's roots.

Physical health, too, can benefit from incremental changes. Consider making modest adjustments to your diet or incorporating short, regular bursts of physical activity. Over time, these small steps can lead to improved overall health, subsequently boosting libido naturally. If coffee is a staple, perhaps switch one cup out for tea. If evenings are sedentary, add a brief walk. Recognise these not as sacrifices, but as investments into a healthier, more vibrant self.

The psychological impact of these slight adjustments should not be underestimated. Each success, no matter how small, contributes to building confidence and self-esteem. This growth makes the journey towards an invigorated sexual relationship less intimidating and more achievable. As you accumulate successes, they reinforce a positive feedback loop, encouraging further change and exploration.

Furthermore, such changes don't necessarily need to be individual. Think about joint activities that you and your partner can embark on together. Shared hobbies or new experiences can introduce fresh energy into your relationship, renewing interest and igniting the spark that's essential to a fulfilling intimate life. These activities remind you both of the companionship and joy that brought you together, rekindling that foundational connection.

In essence, the art of small changes is about reducing the pressure associated with transformation. By shrinking the barriers to action, you're more likely to begin—and sustain—these efforts. Begin with one small change today, and gradually build upon it. Each positive step compounds over time, crafting a new and more harmonious rhythm in both your personal wellness and your shared journey with your partner.

The ripple effect of these gradual improvements can also extend beyond restoring libido. They can enrich multiple dimensions of your life, promoting overall happiness and satisfaction. The aim isn't just the destination, but the confidence and resilience nurtured along the pathway. This journey shapes a future where passion is not merely reignited, but continues to grow and adapt. Remember, meaningful change doesn't always demand a monumental effort; it often starts with the smallest of steps.

## Maintaining Motivation

Motivation can often be an elusive force, especially when you're navigating a journey as personal and intricate as overcoming libido loss. It's a truth universally acknowledged that sustaining motivation requires more than just a fleeting moment of inspiration. You need an underlying, persistent drive. But how do you maintain that drive in the context of cultivating sustainable habits for long-term success in your intimate relationships?

Firstly, it's essential to understand the nature of motivation itself. Motivation isn't a static element that you can 'achieve' once and for all—it's fluid and dynamic, ebbing and flowing with life's circumstances. However, by recognising this fluidity, you can prepare yourself for the inevitability of motivational dips while also celebrating the peaks. Indeed, awareness is your first tool: being mindful of what drives you and when you tend to lose steam can help you preempt these ebbs and strategise accordingly.

To keep motivation alive, start by identifying your personal 'why'. Why are you seeking change? Why is regaining libido significant to you and your relationship? The clearer and more personal your reasons are, the easier it will be to tap into them when you're struggling to keep moving forward. Write these reasons down; make them tangible. Reflect on them regularly, especially during moments of doubt. Knowing your 'why' can be a lighthouse guiding you through the storms of apathy and discouragement.

Another crucial strategy is setting achievable goals. It's tempting to aim high, envisioning a complete transformation overnight. However, if the goals are too grandiose, you're setting yourself up for disappointment. Instead, break down your overarching aim into smaller, manageable milestones. This approach does not only make the journey less daunting but also provides a sense of accomplishment and progress with each step. Achieving these small wins builds momentum, and before you know it, you'll find yourself further along than you'd initially thought possible.

Celebrating these small victories is not to be underestimated. Positive reinforcement plays a huge role in maintaining motivation. When you achieve a milestone, no matter how small, acknowledge it. Celebrate it with your partner. Maybe it's as simple as sticking to a nutritional plan for a week or consistently engaging in open dialogue with your partner. Whatever it is, allow yourself to feel proud. This will create a positive feedback loop, encouraging you to keep going.

Boredom and routine can be motivation killers. When the novelty of a new habit fades, motivation can wane. Counteract this by injecting variety into your journey. If you're trying a new diet for libido enhancement, don't just eat the same meals; experiment with new recipes and flavours. If regular exercise is part of your plan, mix up your routines. Change settings, try new activities, and invite your partner to join you. Not only does this prevent monotony, but it also adds an element of fun and shared experience, enhancing your relationship in the process.

Conversely, there can be too much variety. This might sound contradictory, but while variety keeps things fresh, too much change all at once can overwhelm. It's about finding balance between integrating variety and maintaining consistent routines. Focus on establishing a stable baseline of habits first. Once you've got a rhythm, start adding variety, tweaking one aspect at a time. This gradual approach allows you to enjoy novelty while not derailing the foundation you've laid. Remember, the key to sustainable change is consistency, kissed by creativity.

On this journey, it's also vital to nurture your own sense of self-compassion. Setbacks will happen. There'll be days you fall back into old patterns or feel like progress has stalled. It's important not to let this derail your efforts. Practise self-kindness; treat yourself as you would a dear friend going through a similar situation. Acknowledge the slip without judgment and refocus on your goals, learning from the experience where possible. Every setback is just another stepping stone on your path to lasting change.

Involving your partner can be a tremendous source of motivation. These challenges affect both of you, and working collaboratively can strengthen your bond. Share your goals, your ups and downs. Work through the setbacks together, and celebrate the successes as a team. The mutual support bolsters motivation and cements your relationship. Your partner can be your cheerleader, your sounding board, and most importantly, your confidant in this journey.

Consider the environment as another factor in maintaining motivation. Surround yourself with elements that boost your drive. This could mean decluttering your space, adding reminders and inspiration in your surroundings, or spending time with like-minded people who share similar goals. Reducing barriers—both physical and emotional—can make the journey less burdensome. Don't hesitate to seek out communities or support groups where you can share your journey and hear others' stories. These connections can provide fresh perspectives and renewed motivation.

Lastly, visualisation can be a powerful tool. Imagine how your life and relationship can transform as you work through the stages of reigniting passion and restoring intimacy. Envision the joy, satisfaction, and closeness you'll feel. Take a moment each day to picture this positive outcome as if it's already your reality. This daily practice can boost motivation, grounding it in a vivid, desirable vision of the future.

Maintaining motivation isn't a linear path, but with these strategies, you can thrive in the face of challenges. Remember, motivation is a renewable resource. Each day brings new opportunities to rekindle your drive, reinforcing sustainable habits that pave the way to long-term success in your intimate relationships.

# Chapter 26:
## Reinforcing Intimacy Over Time

Reinforcing intimacy over time in a relationship involves far more than physical connection; it's about nurturing emotional bonds through shared experiences and continued effort. As time passes, keeping the spark alive demands a conscious commitment from both partners. Engaging in shared activities cultivates a sense of partnership and rejuvenates the collective energy within the relationship. Whether it's trying a new hobby, embarking on travel adventures, or simply dedicating time for uninterrupted conversation, these pursuits encourage growth and understanding. Moreover, intertwining interests can deepen bonds and open new avenues for emotional and intellectual intimacy. Continuous relationship building is vital—frequent gestures of appreciation, maintaining open lines of communication, and addressing conflicts constructively can fortify a relationship, making it resilient to the challenges of time. By embracing these principles, couples can craft a bond that evolves gracefully and withstands the test of time, transforming routine into rhythm and companionship into lifelong partnership.

### Keeping the Spark Alive

One of the most cherished aspects of any intimate relationship is the initial spark. However, as time unfolds, many find that the fiery passion they once experienced can diminish. This doesn't signify an end, but a call to action. Keeping the spark alive in a long-term relationship requires intentionality and effort, rooted in a deep understanding of one's partner and oneself. Intimacy, while often perceived as spontaneous, thrives with a little planning and a lot of care.

Consider the role of novelty in relationships. Introducing freshness doesn't mean drastic changes; instead, it involves rediscovering each other's quirks, interests, and desires. It's about creating moments that take you back to when everything felt new. Maybe it's a trip down memory lane, revisiting the place where you first met or sharing tales from the early days. Sometimes, novelty means breaking from routine to try something entirely different, like taking up a new hobby together.

Intimacy also flourishes when partners feel appreciated and seen. Genuine acknowledgment of each other's efforts—whether big or small—can work wonders. Compliments, words of affirmation, and simple gestures of gratitude create an environment where affection can grow naturally. It's about extending appreciation beyond words, making it evident in actions that say, "I see you, and you matter to me."

Furthermore, laughter serves as a delightful conduit to keeping the spark alive. Shared laughter builds a connection that few other things can. Humour can ease tension, reduce stress, and bring partners closer in even the most challenging times. Engaging in activities that invoke laughter—watching a comedy, playing games, or simply being silly together—can remind you why you enjoy each other's company.

Another key element is physical touch, which remains a crucial part of maintaining intimacy. Holding hands, cuddling, or a simple touch on the back as you walk by can reignite that initial flame. Touch transcends verbal communication, offering assurance and warmth. Setting aside time specifically for physical closeness without expectations of leading to more can actually deepen emotional bonds.

Adventure isn't just found in far-off destinations; it's also in the shared journey of life. Embracing adventures—whether they're grand such as travel or subtle like learning a new skill together—adds layers to your shared experiences. These shared challenges and triumphs provide stories that become the fabric of enduring intimacy.

Communication, the linchpin of any relationship, evolves as relationships mature. Delving deeper into conversations about dreams, fears, and desires can refresh understanding and reignite fascination. Sometimes revisiting the basics of effective communication—listening actively, responding thoughtfully, and asking meaningful questions— can rejuvenate a stagnant dynamic.

For some, rituals provide a foundation to build upon. These don't need to be elaborate; a weekly date night, a morning coffee chat, or a dedicated time at the end of the day to connect can be incredibly meaningful. Such rituals become a sanctuary in the chaos of life, rooting partners in their commitment and affection.

Being open to vulnerability with one's partner is another method to maintain a vibrant connection. Allowing yourself to be seen as you truly are, flaws and all, fosters profound intimacy. Being vulnerable embraces authenticity and ushers in a space where partners can feel safe and supported.

Moreover, self-care indirectly contributes to relationship vitality. When individuals take time to nurture themselves, they bring their best selves into the relationship. Whether it's through pursuing personal interests, engaging in solo rejuvenation practices, or seeking professional support when needed, self-care revitalises both partners.

Reflecting on shared goals can help keep the fire burning too. Working towards common aspirations, be they related to personal growth, finances, or family, reinforces the partnership and aligns paths.

This shared focus not only strengthens bonds but also provides a sense of forward momentum.

Naturally, addressing conflicts constructively is crucial. Viewing disagreements as opportunities for growth rather than as threats can transform challenges into means of reinforcing the relationship. Couples who master the art of resolving conflicts with empathy and understanding often emerge stronger and more connected.

Finally, it's important to celebrate achievements, no matter how small. Celebrations create joy and vitality; they remind partners of their capabilities and shared victories. Whether it's an anniversary, a personal achievement, or just making it through another week, these moments reinvigorate the partnership.

In essence, keeping the spark alive isn't about recapturing what once was; it's about creating something even more beautiful. It's an ongoing journey of rediscovery, a dance that marries the familiar with the novel. As you nurture the flame of your relationship, you're not merely keeping it alive; you're letting it forge a more resilient and profound connection over time.

## Shared Activities and Interests

In the ever-evolving landscape of relationships, shared activities and interests can often serve as the glue that holds everything together. When it comes to reigniting intimacy and sustaining it over time, engaging in activities both partners enjoy can be incredibly beneficial. This isn't simply about finding something to pass the time but about genuinely connecting on a deeper level, rekindling the spark that might've dimmed, and nurturing a sense of partnership.

Now, if we delve into the heart of shared activities, the emphasis should be on collaboration and mutual enjoyment. This goes beyond sharing the occasional stroll or watching a film. It's about cultivating shared hobbies or even learning something new together. Think of it as an adventure that adds excitement and a fresh dynamic to the relationship. Whether it's taking up a new sport, cooking exotic recipes, or even attending a dance class, these activities allow couples to explore new facets of themselves and each other.

But why are these shared experiences so crucial? At its core, sharing interests helps ignite a connection that's based on fun, discovery, and sometimes a little healthy competition. Activities that encourage cooperation can introduce a new layer of communication, sparking dialogues that might not arise in everyday conversations. This kind of interaction fosters a greater understanding and appreciation for each other's skills, preferences, and potentially quirky nuances, deepening the bond you share.

Shared activities can also act as a buffer during challenging times. When tensions rise, having an outlet that you both enjoy can redirect energy toward something positive. It's about building resilience in the relationship, knowing there's a common ground you can return to. Let's not forget, laughter is often said to be the best medicine—and sharing a laugh over a failed attempt at a new hobby can be just as bonding as mastering it together.

However, it's important to note that not every activity will work for every couple. Some might find thrill in exploring the outdoors, while others might relish quiet nights in with a new board game. The key is to find what resonates with both partners. Experimentation could be the order of the day; trying a variety of activities until you find those that feel authentic and enriching to your relationship.

There's an added benefit to exploring new interests—personal growth. As individuals within a relationship, pursuing diverse activities allows each person to grow, learn and expand their horizons. This individual enrichment can feed back into the partnership, offering fresher perspectives and newfound excitement to share with each other, keeping the dynamic vibrant and engaging.

In relationships where sexual desire might have waned, shared activities can reignite passion by strengthening emotional intimacy. Passion isn't just about the physical realm—it stems from emotional closeness, mutual understanding, and shared goals. When partners engage in activities that require teamwork, communication, and trust, it can translate into other aspects of their relationship, including the bedroom.

Certain shared activities allow for non-verbal communication, which can be powerful. Dance, for instance, involves a degree of trust and non-verbal cues, encouraging partners to 'speak' to one another through movement and rhythm. Such activities can enhance each partner's ability to tune into physical and emotional cues, eventually translating into other areas of intimacy.

Balancing individual pursuits with shared activities is equally important. While it is crucial to develop shared interests, maintaining a sense of individuality ensures that each partner brings something unique and enriching to the table. It's about nurturing a relationship that thrives on both shared experiences and individual growth, a delicate yet rewarding balance that reinforces intimacy without stifling personal aspirations.

For couples seeking to reignite or reinforce intimacy, creating rituals around shared interests can be incredibly powerful. Be it a weekly game night, designated 'curiosity days' where you explore something new, or simple routines like morning walks, these rituals provide a sense of consistency and predictability that many find comforting. Over time, these rituals become cherished traditions, writing memories into the narrative of your shared lives.

The journey of sharing activities also provides opportunities to reflect on what brought you together in the first place. Was it a shared love for a particular band, a mutual obsession with art, or perhaps a sport you both can't live without? Reviving these initial interests can be a gentle reminder of the foundation from which your relationship has grown, alongside promoting the constant evolution and adaptation that long-term relationships require.

To sum it up, shared activities and interests aren't just a means to fill time—they're essential building blocks in reinforcing intimacy over time. Through fun, creativity, and sometimes challenge, they offer a playground for connection and the opportunity to learn continually more about each other, ensuring that the relationship continues to flourish and evolve. By investing in such pursuits, couples can ignite not just passion but a deeper, more enduring love that continues to enrich their lives together.

## Continuous Relationship Building

Building a continuous and nurturing relationship is much like tending a garden. It requires ongoing attention, occasional adjustments, and a heartfelt commitment to growth. Over time, these conscious efforts sow seeds of intimacy and trust that form the foundation of a passionate romantic partnership. As life's complexities and diversities unfold, keeping this foundation strong demands both partners invest in the relationship with intention and empathy.

Often, the initial excitement and allure that spark a relationship can wane as familiarity settles in. It's not unusual for couples to experience shifts in their emotional and physical connections. Life's evolving responsibilities, from professional pressures to familial commitments, can sometimes overshadow the essential bond of the partnership. Understanding this ebb and flow is vital. Rather than signalling a decline, it can be seen as an invitation to deepen the relationship through continuous and dynamic interaction.

A practical approach to continuous relationship building is maintaining open channels of communication. This might seem like a simple solution, yet its implementation is profoundly impactful. Regular conversations, whether about daily occurrences or profound life changes, help couples stay aligned with each other's thoughts and feelings. By prioritising conversations, couples create a space where honesty and vulnerability are welcome, making it easier to address concerns and celebrate successes together.

Spending quality time together is another pillar of reinforcing intimacy. While hectic schedules can make this challenging, even small, intentional moments can strengthen the relationship. Whether it's having breakfast together without screens, enjoying a leisurely walk in the park, or setting a day for a shared hobby, these moments offer the chance to connect and create memories beyond the mundane rhythm of daily life. Such activities not only rejuvenate the bond but also affirm the value each partner holds in the other's heart.

Physical intimacy is a crucial, yet often overlooked, component of continuous relationship building. It extends beyond sexual connection, enveloping touch, warmth, and closeness in its embrace. Regular acts of affection, like holding hands, hugging, or kissing, reinforce the emotional ties that bind partners together. This physical communication can serve as a reminder of the love and care that underpin the relationship, particularly during testing times.

Trust forms the backbone of any lasting relationship, and building it continuously requires consistent effort and reliable actions. Being faithful to promises, showing up for each other, and maintaining a sense of reliability boosts trustworthiness. It's about demonstrating that both partners are allies, unwavering in support and understanding. This assurance can counteract any external pressures, consolidating the couple's resilience against the strains of life.

Equally important is the ability to adapt and grow individually and as a couple. Relationships are not static; they evolve as both partners change over time. Embracing this evolution requires an open mindset, where each person accepts their own growth as well as their partner's. This perspective not only enriches the relationship but also cultivates a shared vision for the future. Couples who recognise and support each other's aspirations often find a deeper connection as they journey through new levels of understanding and cooperation.

Joint decision-making is another valuable aspect of continuous relationship building. Whether it's choosing a holiday destination or planning for future goals, sharing decisions affirms partnership equality. It encourages a sense of belonging and reinforces that both voices are valued equally. When partners collaborate in decision-making, it fosters a team mentality, where individual interests are respected but mutual happiness is prioritised.

Moreover, resolving conflicts constructively strengthens a relationship over time. It's crucial to remember that disagreements are a natural component of any close relationship. However, navigating these moments with patience and respect can significantly improve relationship satisfaction. Focus on active listening, clear communication of needs, and a willingness to forgive – these strategies ensure that conflicts become stepping stones for growth rather than roadblocks.

Creating rituals and traditions unique to the partnership also plays a critical part in continuous relationship building. Whether it's an annual anniversary getaway or a routine weekly date night, these rituals provide a sense of stability and anticipation. They become cherished anchors that partners can look forward to, offering not only moments of connection but also a shared history that grows with each passing year.

It's also advantageous for couples to engage in joint learning experiences. Whether it's taking up a new language, learning to cook a new cuisine, or attending workshops on mutual interests, exploring new territories together invigorates the relationship with fun and novelty. These activities challenge partners to step out of their comfort zones, revealing new facets of each other, and igniting a spark of adventure in the process.

Lastly, nurturing a sense of gratitude and appreciation is a transformative habit. Acknowledging the efforts, qualities, and gestures that each brings to the relationship reinforces positive feelings and affirms the bond. Regular expressions of gratitude, whether through words or small tokens of affection, encourage partners to view the relationship through a lens of positivity and affection, perpetuating a cycle of kindness and encouragement.

In essence, continuous relationship building is an ongoing journey that requires dedication, creativity, and empathy. By nurturing a supportive and evolving connection, couples can not only maintain but indeed enhance their intimacy over time. Through active engagement and mutual respect, partners can navigate life's dynamics gracefully, ensuring that their relationship remains a vibrant and integral part of their shared existence.

# Conclusion

The journey of understanding and overcoming a decline in libido is a deeply personal one, touching on various facets of life from physical health to emotional wellbeing. As we've explored throughout this book, these challenges are not insurmountable, and the potential for growth and revitalisation is significant. By now, it should be clear that the loss of sexual desire can be attributed to a tapestry of causes, and in recognising this complexity, opportunities for meaningful and effective change become possible.

At the heart of rejuvenating one's sexual desire is a commitment to self-awareness and openness. Embracing the discussions on hormonal influences and psychological factors offers a foundational step towards identifying the unique contributors to your experience. Understanding how these elements interplay with personal identity and lifestyle enables a clearer vision of the changes and adaptations required to foster improvement.

It cannot be overstated just how critical the role of communication is within relationships. Open dialogue about libido changes not only supports finding solutions but also strengthens the relational bond. Emotional closeness and trust grow from these conversations, paving the way for joint exploration in creating new, exciting experiences that rekindle passion. Partners can become invaluable allies, working together to not just restore but enhance intimacy.

The necessity of a balanced lifestyle is another pivotal piece of this puzzle. Consistent exercise, nutritious eating, and adequate rest lay the groundwork for physical health that underpins libido. These aren't just isolated activities; they're interconnected practices that nurture the body and mind. By focusing on these areas, you can significantly impact not just sexual health but overall wellbeing, creating a synergy that supports sustained vitality. Furthermore, mindfulness techniques offer another layer of depth, cultivating a mind-body connection that enhances intimate experiences and reduces stress, a known deterrent to desire.

Yet, there's also great value in understanding and embracing alternative approaches, including therapeutic options and medical treatments, which can provide customised solutions for specific challenges. Whether through professional counselling or incorporating new health practices like vitamins and supplements, these strategies can enhance the effectiveness of broader efforts, allowing for a tailored approach that respects individuality.

In the context of aging, adjusting expectations and welcoming the shifts that come with it offer opportunities for growth rather than decline. This perspective encourages embracing how desire might evolve and recognising that each stage of life can offer new dimensions of pleasure and connection.

Moreover, the impact of external influences such as media can shape perceptions of libido and masculinity, often unhelpfully. By critically evaluating these messages and cultivating a more balanced view, you create a space that respects reality over myth, emphasising personal experience over societal standards.

No less important is the power of small, sustainable changes. Long-term success stems from developing routines that become second nature, reinforcing positive changes in a gradual yet consistent manner. Celebrating even small victories nurtures motivation, transforming a transient triumph into a lasting habit that supports ongoing libido health.

Ultimately, reigniting desire and deepening intimacy isn't a singular destination but rather a continuous journey enriched by an adventurous spirit and a commitment to growth. The capacity for renewal exists within each individual; it's a matter of recognising and cultivating it. Through awareness, communication, and action, you can draw closer to a life that's not only rich in passion but also in genuine human connection.

In conclusion, this book serves as both a guide and a companion, offering insights and strategies aligned with your unique needs and desires. The pursuit of understanding libido loss and rekindling passion is deeply transformative, and this transformation can bring not only personal fulfillment but also a more profound and satisfying connection with your partner. As you move forward, may the knowledge and insights gained here support you in creating a relationship filled with intimacy, trust, and enduring passion.

# Appendix A:
# Appendix

The appendix serves as a crucial extension of our exploration, offering additional layers of context and support to the core topics previously discussed. It's meant to be both a resource and a companion, filled with insights that have the potential to transform how you approach the challenges detailed in the book and the solutions we've proposed.

In this section, you won't find basic repetitions of what we've already covered. Instead, you'll discover a collection of supplementary materials, practical tools, and insightful perspectives, all designed to enrich your journey towards revitalising intimacy and passion. While each chapter provided foundational knowledge and strategies, the appendix acts as a bridge, carrying the conversation further and grounding it in practicality.

First, we've included an assortment of practical exercises and self-assessment tools. These have been carefully crafted to empower you to introspect and evaluate your personal experiences, helping to translate theory into meaningful personal growth. By engaging with these activities, you have the opportunity to tailor the insights of the book to your unique circumstances, fostering a more personalised journey of rediscovery.

Moreover, you'll find thoughtful reflections from partners who have walked this path. These narratives provide a dual perspective, offering partners a voice and adding depth to the understanding of shared experiences. Acknowledging the stories of others can open up new avenues for empathy and mutual recognition, reinforcing the relational elements discussed in the chapters.

We also present a curated selection of recommended readings and resources. These have been chosen to enhance your understanding of the multifaceted aspects of libido, intimacy, and relationship dynamics. Engaging with these resources can widen your lens, providing you with fresh insights and contemporary thinking in the field.

Lastly, the appendix concludes with a compendium of frequently asked questions and their detailed responses. Structured to anticipate your most pressing concerns, these FAQs are designed to give you clear, concise, and actionable answers. Whether you're grappling with a specific issue or seeking clarity on a nuanced topic, this section stands ready to assist.

As we conclude, remember that the appendix is more than a supplement; it's an invitation to continue exploring, questioning, and growing. By engaging with these resources, you equip yourself with the means to sustain the momentum built throughout the book. Here's to taking those next steps with confidence and renewed vigour.

www.ingramcontent.com/pod-product-compliance
Lightning Source LLC
Chambersburg PA
CBHW022245290526
45785CB00015B/193